# PSYCHIATRIC PEER REVIEW: PRELUDE AND PROMISE

Edited by
John M. Hamilton, M.D.

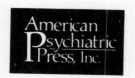

1400 K Street, N.W.
Washington, DC 20005

*To the two Don's and Hank,*
*without whom none of this*
*would make any difference.*

Copyright © 1985 John M. Hamilton
ALL RIGHTS RESERVED
Manufactured in the United States of America

**Library of Congress Cataloging in Publication Data**

Main entry under title:

Psychiatric peer review.

  Includes bibliographies.
  1. Peer review in psychiatry.  2. Peer review in
psychiatry—United States.  3. Psychiatry—Standards—
United States.  I. Hamilton, John M., 1923–
[DNLM:  1. Peer Review.  2. Psychiatry—standards.
WM 21 P9735]
RC455.2.P43P79      1985      362.2      85-13517
ISBN 0-88048-211-7

# Contents

# Contributors

**Daniel B. Borenstein, M.D.**
Assembly Liaison, APA Peer Review Committee;
Private Practice
Los Angeles, California

**Henry A. Davis, M.D.**
Private Practice
San Diego, California

**James Egan, M.D.**
Member, APA Peer Review Committee;
Chairman, Department of Psychiatry
Children's National Medical Center
Washington, D.C.

**William Guillette, M.D.**
Medical Director
Personal Financial Security Division
Aetna Life and Casualty
Hartford, Connecticut

**John Hamilton, M.D.**
Chair, APA Peer Review Committee;
Private Practice
Columbia, Maryland

**Charles F. Marsh, M.D.**
Private Practice
San Diego, California

**Joseph R. Mawhinney, M.D.**
Private Practice
San Diego, California

**Ronald S. Mintz, M.D.**
Member, APA Peer Review Committee;
Private Practice
Los Angeles, California

**William C. Offenkrantz, M.D.**
Member, APA Peer Review Committee;
Professor of Psychoanalysis and Psychiatry
Medical College of Wisconsin
Milwaukee, Wisconsin

**Gary L. Shepherd, M.D.**
Consultant, APA Peer Review Committee;
Private Practice
San Diego, California

**George F. Wilson, M.D.**
Member, APA Peer Review Committee;
President, Carrier Foundation
Belle Mead, New Jersey

# Prelude

Over the last decade, organized medicine in general and psychiatry in particular have taken critical interest in responding to issues related to quality of medical care and medical care cost escalation. As the consumer-at-large and third-party payers have sought to bring about a balance that might be acceptable both to providers and to users of medical services, tensions have developed within our medical care delivery system which we, the professionals, have attempted to ease without destroying that system or disrupting its usefulness to consumers. Peer review is one aspect of quality assurance programming that has taken a significant place in attempting to bring stability to the system, which is very often tenuously balanced.

Peer review was institutionalized in Public Law 92-603, which established the requirement for a system of Professional Standards Review Organizations (PSROs). As identified in the PSRO legislation, peer review is designed to preserve professional self-determination through professional monitoring of utilization, quality, and cost. It seeks to correct problems in practice through careful monitoring, persuasion and education (Tischler and Astrachan 1982).

This book is essentially about the first decade of the American Psychiatric Association's endeavors to involve itself formally in all of the arenas where the professional input of the actively practicing psychiatric provider may produce expertise to enhance care quality while insisting on cost-effectiveness. This book will discuss the history, methodology, problems and concerns, special case implications, and the promise of psychiatry's national effort.

We recognize that this is a rapidly changing field and that by the time this book goes to press some of its content will have become passé. However, a pause to document the experiences thus far in the development of peer review technology is thought to be useful before too much of its early growth and travail might be forgotten.

John M. Hamilton, M.D.


## REFERENCE

Tischler GL, Astrachan BM: Quality Assurance in Mental Health: Peer and Utilization Review. Washington, DC, U.S. Department of Health and Human Services, 1982

# 1

# Quality Assurance in Historical Perspective

*David J. Fine*
*Eve R. Meyer*

# Quality Assurance in Historical Perspective

T here is a temptation in our technocratic age to ascribe most innovation to the near term past. Quality assurance activities in health care are often accorded no history beyond the life breathed into these programs by the Joint Commission on Accreditation of Hospitals in the last two decades. In fact, the issues we presently face in assessing and improving the quality of health care have existed throughout recorded medical history.

## EARLY HISTORY

In Paris' Louvre Museum stands a 7½-foot block of chiseled diorite dating from 2000 B.C. on which is inscribed the cuneiform code of King Hammurabi of Babylon. When the laborious task of deciphering the text was completed, it was found to contain the earliest known listing of charges that could be exacted by a physician (Sigerist 1932; Venzmer 1968). In the same passage, physicians are notified of penalties for incompetent practice:

*If the doctor shall treat a gentleman and shall open an abscess with the knife and shall preserve the eye of the*

Reprinted in revised form by permission from *Hospital Health Services Administration*, Vol. 28, Number 6, November/December 1983.

*patient he shall receive ten shekels of silver. If the doctor
shall open an abscess with a blunt knife and shall kill the
patient or shall destroy the sight of the eye, his hand shall
be cut off (Ackerknecht 1955).*

Quality and cost of medical care, as societal concerns, have
thus been interwined since earliest times.

Artifacts indicating prehistoric medical intervention in
disease exist in sufficient numbers to create paleomedicine
as a distinct field of study. Papyri documenting Egyptian
civilization describe the Egyptian physician's acumen coupled with another characteristic of high-quality medicine:
the need to set forth the state-of-the-art so that others can
practice it accordingly. This has the advantage of allowing
wide dissemination of a set of observations, but the concomitant disadvantage of occasionally endowing those observations with an encrustation of dogma (Stenn 1967).

Perhaps the best known of papyri are the Edwin Smith
Papyrus and the Ebers Papyrus, both of which are approximately 4000 years old. Each is a medical textbook containing case histories, provisional diagnoses, instructions for
examination, prognosis indications, and therapeutic measures, including incantation, manipulation, and medication. The Ebers Papyrus alone contains 876 prescriptions
for drugs, utilizing more than 500 different substances. It
covers conditions as diverse as hematuria, tumors and ar-
thritis (Stenn 1967). The following fragment illustrates the
whole:

*If thou examinest a man for an illness in his cardia, and all
his limbs are heavy for him . . . thou shalt put thy hand
over his cardia, if thou findest his cardia drumming and it
is going and coming under thy fingers, then thou shalt say
about it: it is a weakness of digestion that has prevented
him from eating before.*

*Thou shalt effect all his evacuation for him . . . dates
. . . pulped with beer. . . . If thou examinest him after this
has been done, and thou findest his breast-bone warm and
his belly cool, then thou shalt say: his weakness has gone
down (Ackerknecht 1955).*

The body of knowledge among Egyptian physicians had
grown sufficiently great by the time of Herodotus. The practice of general medicine had given way to specialized ac-

tivity in which a greater degree of knowledge could be applied. The depth, rather than the breadth, of knowledge of the individual physician came to be valued in this civilization as a signal indication of quality. In Herodotus' view:

> The practice of medicine is so divided among them, that each physician is a healer of one disease and no more. All of the country is full of physicians, some of the eye, some of the teeth, some of what pertains to the belly and some of hidden diseases . . . (Venzmer 1968).

Such specialization ended with its host civilization, and did not reappear for another 2000 years.

The situation was quite different when, in the fifth century B.C., the Greeks revered one existing health care system to such a degree that they founded medical schools on the island of Cos to further its use. The school was dedicated to the healing of the whole person, physically and spiritually, and placed a greater value on prognosis than on diagnosis. It has as a deity the demi-god of healing, Aesculapius, to whose spa-like shrines pilgrims traveled for physical and spiritual relief (Venzmer 1968). The school at Cos grew in influence because there was a forceful quality about the ideas presented by its principal teacher, Hippocrates. In time, he came to be the idealized image of the dedicated physician. A special group of Hippocrates' manuscripts are concerned with the legal and ethical obligations of the physician, and certain practical advice regarding conduct that would not bring disgrace on the profession:

> This piece of advice is of importance. Do not begin by worrying the patient about your fee. If you do, you will arouse in the patient a suspicion that unless he agrees to your terms you will go away and leave him to his fate. So do not concentrate your attention on fixing what your fee is to be. A worry of this nature is likely to harm the patient, particularly if the disease be an acute one. Hold fast to reputation rather than profit. It is better to reproach patients you have saved than to distress men who are at death's door (Cope 1957).

One may well ask why Hippocrates went to such lengths to discourage loutish behavior in his followers when no one had done so before him. The answer lies in the atmosphere of theoretical ferment within which he practiced. Instead of having, as in Egypt, a multiplicity of specialties within a single profession, there was a multiplicity of healing professions, of which Hippocratic medicine was simply one of the more prominent. Thus rudeness and exploitation would have to be discouraged in the interests of a favorable public image relative to competitors.

The emphasis on prognosis as a skill was also a product of these competitive circumstances. In the absence of licensure, no means existed by which a physician of the Hippocratic bent could establish himself as a credible practitioner. Hippocrates recognized this, maintaining

> that it is an excellent thing for a physician to practice forecasting. For if he discover and declare unaided by the side of his patients the present, the past, and the future, and fill in the gaps in the account given by the sick, he will be the more believed to understand the cases, so that men will confidently entrust themselves to him for treatment (Sigerist 1941).

The rendering of an accurate prognosis, therefore, was the hallmark of a competent professional.

Hippocrates is popularly known for originating the oath administered to every physician who completed his course of study in that time, a version of which is still used today at many medical graduations. Although actual authorship of the oath is certainly in doubt, its importance lies in the fact that responsibility for its enforcement was placed on the physician himself. He has sworn adherence by the relevant deities and this was his guarantee to his preceptors that the standards of the profession would be maintained as they had been imparted (Etziony 1973).

## UNIFORM PRACTICE ESTABLISHED

The reputation of the Greek physician spread in the narrow circle of organized civilization, particularly in Rome, and the physicians themselves began to disperse along Greece's network of Mediterranean trade routes.

Even though Greek medical skills were generally favored, there was no means of ascertaining fitness among a highly variable assortment of practitioners. The situation must have reached a point of national discomfort because, in the first century A.D., the Emperor Antoninus Pius issued a "numerous clausus" establishing that every city, depending on community size, could have five, seven or ten physicians in practice. These would be the valde docti, the true physicians, and admission to their ranks was dependent on submission of credentials to a common council of the emperor (Sigerist 1932).

The edict is notable in that it addressed both the need for uniform standards of practice and uniform geographical distribution, certain areas having apparently become vastly more preferable to others. Credentials presented as a result of the decree are preserved in papyri from Egypt, testifying to its enforcement throughout the empire (Sigerist 1941).

The synthesizing force in Roman medicine was the Greek physician, Galen of Pergamos. In the second century A.D., peripatetic as his precursors, he arrived in Rome after having studied medicine in various parts of Asia Minor and having served for a time as physician to the gladiators in his hometown. Galen became body physician to the Emperor Marcus Aurelius and during his tenure helped influence the transition of medicine from an art to a science by reporting his observations and anatomical studies in 100 medical treatises filling 22 volumes (Ackerknecht 1955).

Galen, too, sought to upgrade the conduct of the profession—not with the positive prescription of Hippocrates, but with wrathful denunciation of the venality of his contemporaries. For example, of the medical students who wished to cease their studies and begin practicing prematurely in order to earn fees, he wrote:

*The only difference between a robber and a doctor is that the former commits his crimes in the mountains and the latter commits them in Rome (Venzmer 1968).*

The status of physicians was elevated as a result of Galen's efforts, including exemption from taxes, military conscription, and forced relocation to colonies (Venzmer 1968). With a body of documents that recorded medical knowledge in its supposed entirety, the state assumed responsibility for the education and training of physicians, and professors of medicine were appointed in Rome (Sigerist 1941). By the sixth century A.D., a flourishing medical school had been founded in Ravenna.

## GALEN'S THEORIES RESTRICTED PHYSICIANS

Galen's theories on the basic humor of the body, however erroneous, were taught intact and would be for nearly 14 centuries. Where formerly the medical societies of Rome awarded prizes to physicians reporting the finest cure, or inventing the best surgical instrument (Sigerist 1932), the teachings of Galen became a boundary beyond which no physician could pass. This standardization, however, assured some continuance of quality and did the individual practitioner no ill because the profession had become accepted by the public over other healing disciplines. Physicians practiced successfully in a fiercely competitive private market or attached themselves to the wealthy as personal physicians (Sigerist 1941) in a model that continued into Europe's Middle Ages. Galen himself had provided the formula for success:

> If, however, there is anyone who would like to be famous, not just for ingenious speeches but for deeds as well, then all he need do is to absorb without effort what I have spent a whole lifetime of eager research in discovering (Venzmar 1968).

Ironically, his research and its effect on subsequent original inquiry temporarily brought recognized intellectual curiosity in the field of medicine to a halt.

Advancements in medicine were more active in the East after the teachings of Galen became firmly established in Europe. In Persia, the medical profession existed in competition with herbalists and priests. The holy Vendidad recorded the situation at about A.D. 200:

> If several healers offer themselves together, O Spitama Zarathustra, namely, one who heals with the knife, one who heals with herbs, and one who heals with the holy

*work, it is this last who will best drive away sickness from the body of the faithful (Wilcocks 1965).*

Persian physicians had not yet, in other words, established a monopoly among healing arts.

At its height, Persian medicine was dominated by Avicenna, who synthesized Greek and Arabic medicine into a comprehensive system of medical science. By the time of his death A.D. 1037, the medical profession had blossomed among the far-flung possessions of the Caliphs. Here, too, assuring quality became a problem. Caliph al-Muqtadir took the situation in hand by issuing a proclamation specifying that no one could practice medicine in Baghdad unless he had been examined by the physician Sinan ibn Thabit of Harran (Sigerist 1935) and, effectively, license to do so had been issued.

There is a fundamental difference between this edict and that of Rome's Antoninus Pius. The Caliph required, for the first time, that all practitioners of healing arts undergo an examination. Antoninus, by contrast, had certified that the five to seven doctors assigned to a city were worthy, without putting restrictions on other healers. Residents of Baghdad, on the other hand, could be assured that any physician they consulted had passed the test. Other Persians were presumably not so fortunate, and the consumer-oriented standards contained in the doctrines of the holy Avesta were the best standard of practice available.

These doctrines offered a pragmatic emphasis on the outcome of treatment as the standard of care, and stated: "if he treat with the knife for the third time a worshipper of the Daevas and he die, he is unfit to practice the art of healing forever and ever" (Sigerist 1941). This may be contrasted to the professional qualifications preferred by the Caliph. The controversy regarding judgments of outcome, as opposed to credentials and qualifications, exists to this day.

A separate art of healing developed in China, more or less contemporaneously with its Mediterranean counterparts. Documents from the Chou Dynasty period (1122–221 B.C.) indicate that each physician was required to pass a state examination before entering practice, and professional regulation was "definitely a part of the government's business" (Veith 1943; Venzmer 1968). Rather than limiting itself to this professional credentialing mechanism, the government sought, like the Persians, to measure the physician's worth by the outcome of his patients. This was accomplished administratively instead of leaving the process to the experiences of the consumer.

Chou Li, or Rites of Chou, an administrative document written during the Chou Dynasty, describes the system:

> The chief physician is in charge of the regulation of the medicines and all the drugs which are used in order to render medical services. All those in the administration of the empire who are ill and those who have colics and ulcers come to him for treatment. Furthermore he charges the physicians with the individual care and the curing of the patients. At the end of the year he examines the work of these physicians in order to determine their subsistence. Ten completed treatments make a first-rate superior physician. Next in line come those who have made one error in 10 treatments; then those who have made two errors in 10 treatments; and those who have made four errors in 10 treatments make second-rate inferior physicians (Veith 1943).

What makes this passage particularly notable is the statement "to determine their subsistence." Physicians were dependent on the judgment rendered for the rate at which they would be reimbursed for practicing their livelihood.

## THE MIDDLE AGES

In the tenth century, the physician Constantine of Africa ended nearly 40 years of travel through the known world by settling into monastic life at Monte Cassino. He brought copies of the ancient Greek and Roman medical classics, preserved in Arabic, which he translated into Latin (Venzmer 1968). The arts thus transcribed were readily applied at Monte Cassino, where medical treatment was a church function.

The effects of the translation were felt almost immediately with the founding of the West's oldest medical school at nearby Salerno. During the next two centuries, centers of learning were established at Paris, Montpellier, Toledo, Bologna, Oxford and Padua (Ackerknecht 1955). The works of Galen formed the core of the curriculum, and the schools were the nucleus of the medical profession. Moreover, they provided a reference point in establishing the quality of care. The Norman King, Roger, issued the following proclamation in the mid-1100s:

> *Who, from now on, wishes to practice medicine, has to present himself before our officials and examiners, in order to pass their judgment. Should he be bold enough to disregard this, he will be punished by imprisonment and confiscation of his entire property. In this way we are taking care that our subjects are not endangered by the inexperience of the physicians. Nobody dare practice medicine unless he has been found fit by the convention of the Salernitan masters (Sigerist 1935).*

The teachings of Galen were imparted intact. Anatomical inaccuracies went unnoticed because surgery was a separate field practiced largely by barbers and the church forbade dissection of a human. Nevertheless, the body of knowledge was so respected that by the middle of the next century, the Emperor Frederick II of Hohenstaufen issued a credentials-oriented edict similar to the Norman law, which required three years' study of logic and humanities followed by five years of medical courses and an examination (Sigerist 1935).

The physician was again being judged on his credentials, but now the criteria were not what he knew, but what he had been taught. This philosophical inversion notwithstanding, the medical faculties assumed increasing importance in the process of "licensure" and they became more strongly influenced by the church. Special arrangements were made by Jewish physicians, who could not be licensed by a representative of the Pope and were therefore directly licensed by the medical faculty (Sigerist 1935). Strict and binding fee tariffs were once again set for physicians, this time by the medical faculties (Sigerist 1941).

## THE RENAISSANCE

In the fourteenth and fifteenth centuries, a series of plagues ravaged Europe. Medical science, as it then existed, was powerless to combat them and was, moreover, reluctant to try. As an aftermath, most of the sturdy doctrines of the Middle Ages, including the teachings of Galen, were rendered obsolete.

Andreas van Wesele, a young Belgian medical student, Latinized his name to Vesalius, as was the fashion of the time, when he began to attend the University of Paris medical school. He abandoned the teachings of Galen and began a sinister self-education: during the night he unearthed recently buried corpses and dissected them in secret. He concluded from these efforts that Galen had never dissected a human body. Disillusioned, he returned to Louvain, and at the age of 21 received permission to dissect corpses and give anatomical lectures. He aroused the interest of the Inquisition by these activities and fled to Padua.

After only a few months there, he was awarded a Doctor of Medicine degree and on the following day, at the age of 23, was appointed professor of anatomy and surgery. With a young artist to record each step in woodcuts, Vesalius performed dissection and wrote a seven-volume encyclopedia of human anatomy published at Basle in 1543. The obstinate reign of Galen was decisively shaken.

Vesalius' work was received with derision by the conservative medical faculties, and his own professor at Paris openly referred to him as "Vesanus" or "madman." The same man coined an ingenious explanation for the contradictions with Galen: the human body had undoubtedly changed since the time of Galen. In particular, the different curvature of femur was due to the fashion of wearing narrow trousers. Vesalius, hounded and discouraged, retired from research to become court physician to the Spanish king and died following a shipwreck while on a pilgrimage to the Holy Land (Ackerknecht 1955; Stenn 1967).

The medieval faculties responded slowly to the abrupt changes taking place within the medical profession. By hesitating, they lost power over regulation of physicians to the state, and each town to which a physician moved was entitled to subject him to an examination of credentials (Sigerist 1935). Moreover, he was frequently required by civil authorities to take an oath of service as in the "Oath of Doctor and Physician in the Town of Ambers":

*[Likewise] he shall swear that he shall take care of and treat all the sick consulting him to the best of his ability. He*

*shall not prepare any drugs himself; . . . he should not charge more for them than what is paid for them in the pharmacy. He shall not charge the citizens more for any herb than what he paid for it himself; the profit he takes shall be just and modest. He shall not be out of town overnight without consent of a councillor or the mayor himself (Etziony 1973).*

The restrictions placed on the practice of the physician, and the protection afforded the rights of the apothecary, indicate that apothecaries were organized as a profession, whereas physicians still functioned as entrepreneurs. This was, however, an era in which all professions were forming societies that, among other services, would intercede with civil authorities.

## EARLY PROFESSIONAL SELF-REGULATION

In England, for example, during the reign of Henry VII, three surgeons were tried before the mayor of London on charges of incompetent treatment of a hand wound. A group of fellow surgeons acted as arbitrators in an early example of peer review. They gained the acquittal of the accused surgeons by arguing that the wound had been treated with "the moon remaining in the sign Gemini," but that cautery had saved the patient's life (Wilcocks 1965).

With such examples of professional self-regulation, the Royal College of Physicians was founded in 1518 during the reign of King Henry. Its avowed purpose was

*to curb the audacity of those wicked men who shall profess medicine more for the sake of their avarice than from the assurance of any good conscience, whereby very many inconveniences may ensue to the rude and credulous populace (Wilcocks 1965).*

This group of eight physicians assumed licensure control of all physicians practicing within a 7-mile radius of London. As in the days of the Caliphs, the practitioners, not the medical faculties or the civilian authorities, assessed credentials. Outside this geographic boundary, licensure remained in the hands of the Church of England (Raach 1943).

The Royal College of Physicians was not the first licensing mechanism in Europe. The faculty at the University of Paris had undertaken, in the fourteenth century, a licensure effort so drastic that it resembled an inquisition. Vowing to stamp out charlatanism and quackery, the faculty, with support from church authorities, conducted trials of unlicensed practitioners. While some outright thievery may have been prevented, efforts were typically directed at persons who conducted healing activities without the benefit of a diploma from a university. Special attention was given to removing women from the healing arts, under the ingenious argument that they were already barred from practicing law because of their ignorance and could do far greater damage to the physical body if allowed to practice medicine (Kibre 1953).

Physicians, apothecaries, and barber-surgeons practiced independently of one another, even during the heyday of the Faculty of Paris (Kibre 1953), and they still did so in sixteenth-century London. While physicians directed the activities of the apothecary with respect to their own patients, many apothecaries also undertook to diagnose and prescribe on their own, which found an immense popularity with the majority of the people who could not afford care by a physician. This was resented by physicians, but they made no effort to intervene (Wilcocks 1965). Furthermore, the Royal College did not seek to prevent all the unlicensed from practice, and a 1604 license indicated among the qualifications, "had already effected notable cures" (Nagel 1934).

The Royal College was extraordinarily active during its earliest days, dividing its activities into distinct academic, administrative and medico-political spheres. Its academic functions included teaching and examining students. Administratively, it enforced licensure and adherence to ethics. These two areas had already received attention from previous organizations. Medico-political activities, however, comprised a totally new arena. Members of the Royal College also advised the government, the universities, corporations, and the general public on aspects of health.

In 1858, the English government introduced a Medical Care Act, which provided a common basis for the training and registration of medical practitioners. Power to do so was solely in the hands of the government, and the regulatory reign of the Royal College ended (McLachlan and McKeown 1971).

## AMERICAN COLONIAL PERIOD

In 1639, the New World's first piece of medical legislation was enacted in Virginia. Its wording indicates that the profession was becoming established in the settlements, and also that settlers themselves wished to exert their own resilient influence on it:

> . . . consideration being had and taken of the immoderate and excessive rates and prices exacted by practitioners in physick and chyryrgery. . . . It was therefore enacted for the better redress of the like abuses . . . the regulating [of] phisitians and chirurgeons within the collony, That it should be lawfull and free for any person or persons in such cases where they should conceive the acco't of the phisitian or chirurgeon to be unreasonable either for his pains or for his druggs or medicines, to arrest the said phisitian or chirurgeon either to the quarter court or county court where they inhabitt . . . and it was further ordered that when it should be sufficiently proved in any of the said courts that a phisitian or chirurgeon had neglected his patient, or that he had refused . . . his helpe and assistance to any person or persons in sickness or extremity, That the phisitian or chirurgeon should be censured by the said court for . . . his neglect or refuseal . . . (Gordon 1949).

This act placed regulation of the physician in the hands of local magistrates and juries. It was passed at the same time that the Royal College of Physicians was in its heyday in England and the Faculty of Paris held sway over France. A physician's relocation to the New World, therefore, meant a return to the days before self-regulation. As the population of the North American continent increased, however, the law of supply and demand must have exerted an influence on the Virginia Assembly. In 1660, it added a mollifying amendment that entitled the physician to collect his fee from patients:

*for meanes administered and paines taken in the fitt of*
*sickness whereof the patient dyes, and where the patient*
*recovers six months after such recovery and noe longer*
*(Gordon 1949).*

Politics and the practice of medicine went hand in
hand. Not only were the politician and the physician frequently one and the same, but the practice of medicine was
forced to adapt itself to the legislative body by which it was
controlled. Lacking in European tradition and unopposed
by any professional organization, legislators were free to try
whatever approach to medical regulation they wished. In
1670, Massachusetts enacted regulations resembling those
of Virginia, but added a clause that specifically prohibited
the use of remedies not generally accepted as tried and true.
The clause further stipulated that any radical or violent
form of treatment could only be undertaken with the patient's consent, and not without consultation by medical
experts or other knowledgeable persons (Duffy 1976; Kett
1968; Nagel 1934).

## PROHIBITIVE LICENSURE

Thus, in one generation, from the time physicians were
first made answerable to the local political structure, issues
of consent, required consultation and human investigation
had been raised. A century before the Declaration of Independence was signed, an indelible stamp was placed on the
character of American medicine. Oddly, licensure lagged
behind these measures. In the 1650s, colonial legislatures
began issuing licenses to individual practitioners, but did
not prohibit the unlicensed from practicing (Kett 1968).

The first form of prohibitive licensure was directed
against ships' surgeons seeking to practice on land, and
required them to obtain legislative license first. Since ships'
surgeons were highly esteemed, the measure was not directed at quality control as much as at prevention of competition (Nagel 1934). By the close of the seventeenth century, the distinction between physicians, surgeons, and
apothecaries blurred and practitioners known as "empirics"
appeared, swelling the ranks of healers in the hinterlands.

A catalytic factor in the establishment of professional identity in the New World was legislation enacted in Virginia in 1736. This statute set a general schedule of fees for services performed by a "practicer of phisic." Interestingly, these were calculated by using the number of miles traveled by the physician with a surcharge permitted for "those persons who have studied phisic in any university, and taken any degree therein . . . " (Gordon 1949).

For the first time, a differentiation between the educated and the uneducated physician was drawn. Moreover, the educated physician was to be reimbursed at a greater rate. Young medical practitioners who possessed the wealth began to seek medical education abroad to qualify for the higher status a university degree afforded. While studying abroad, chiefly in Edinburgh and Leyden, they were exposed to European licensure systems and the critical role played by professional organizations and university faculties. The European-educated physician began to feel a sense of his own superiority, and kinship to his educated colleagues.

In 1744 Dr. Alexander Hamilton wrote derisively of an empiric,

> He had been a shoemaker in town and was a notable fellow at his trade, but happening two years agoe to cure an old woman of a pestilential mortal disease, he thereby acquired the character of a physitian, was applied to from all quarters, and finding the practice of physick a more profitable business than cobling, he laid aside his awls and leather, got himself some gallipots, and instead of cobling of soals, fell to cobling of human bodies (Kett 1968).

By 1757, William Smith wrote in his "History of New York,"

> Few physicians among us are eminent for their skill. Quacks abound like locusts in Egypt, and too many have recommended themselves to a full and profitable practice and subsistence. This is the less to be wondered at, as the profession is under no kind of regulation. Loud as the call is, to our shame be it remembered we have no law to protect the lives of the King's subjects from the malpractice of pretenders. Any man at his pleasure sets up for physician, apothecary, and chirurgeon. No candidates are either ex-

*amined or licensed, or even sworn for fair practice (Gordon
1949).*

## EARLY AMERICAN LICENSURE ACTS

In 1760, New York enacted the first exclusive licensure act,
which provided that no one practice medicine or surgery
without being examined or licensed by a government-ap-
pointed board of examiners. New Jersey followed in 1772
with a licensure act requiring physicians to pass an examination conducted by two judges of the Supreme Court
(Bordley and Harvey 1976). Other legislatures followed suit,
but some states, poorer and more sparsely doctored, did not
enact licensure requirements until the 1830s (Kett 1968).

A tentative introduction of the European system had
been established, but it lacked two critical elements in existence in Europe: medical schools and medical societies.
Prototypes of these appeared briefly in the mid-1700s, affiliated with the Pennsylvania Hospital, but the Revolution
subsequently preoccupied the medical profession.

At the end of the Revolutionary War, there were about
3,500 healing practitioners in the United States (Bell 1975).
"Regular" physicians were outnumbered by apprenticed or
domestic practitioners by a ratio of ten to one. The former
tended to cluster in larger cities where the impetus to organize lay almost completely with the educated physicians
who had been exposed to professional societies during their
European studies. The desirability of forming an all-in-
clusive society that would allow for control of uneducated
physicians from within, or the creation of an exclusive
organization to exert external political control over the uneducated, was debated, with the former course of action
being selected.

## ELITE MEDICAL SOCIETIES

Prototypical medical societies that were little more than
debating societies that published occasional papers had
existed earlier. But in 1780 the Boston society was re-
organized along restrictive lines, designed to include only
the wealthiest and most influential practitioners. These

were the persons most likely to benefit from mutual consultation and elimination of competition. The organization's charter limited its membership to 70 (Kett 1968).

In Philadelphia and New York, new organizations emulated this elite model. Measures to distinguish between approved and unapproved physicians were fairly informal and limited to testimonial letters regarding competence. It was hoped that membership in the organization would, in and of itself, become a symbol of competence, and this did occur. The founders of the Boston Medical Society served as the city's quarantine officers, and the New York Society recommended surgeons to the army and navy. By 1800, 10 local medical societies and 5 state medical societies were in existence, primarily in the northeast and mid-Atlantic states (Rothstein 1972).

Early American licensure systems lacked many of the elements of European legislation. No sanctions of appreciable magnitude were leveled against the unlicensed, no uniform standards were established, and no professional organization stood ready to separate the competent from the unworthy. The science of medicine was considered to be so rudimentary that lay persons would not have found its technology beyond their understanding, and could therefore be expected to make competency distinctions themselves.

New York amended its licensure act in 1797 to stipulate educational qualifications and levied a $25 fine for conducting unlicensed practice (Davis 1903). Five other state societies (Massachusetts, New Hampshire, Connecticut, Maryland, and Rhode Island) did likewise, viewing licensure authority as their major field of activity (Rothstein 1972). In the main, such statutes simply entitled licensed physicians to sue for debts, and therefore only prevented the unlicensed from so suing. Special practitioner categories such as midwives and apothecaries were often specially exempted from licensure.

The populist values of the Jacksonian period in the 1830s saw repeal of many hard-won licensure measures because of adverse public reaction to the harsh therapeutic measures employed by physicians and the public's demand for freedom of choice (Rothstein 1972). Organized medicine learned that licensure, as a discrediting mechanism, was effective only against the aberrant individual and was powerless when confronted with popular movements such as Thomsonian Herbalism and Homeopathic practice, first brought to America in 1825.

One of the early crusaders for academic preparation of reputable practitioners through medical education was Dr. Daniel Drake. Born to impoverished Kentucky settlers and educated in a one-room school, he was apprenticed to a physician at the age of 15 (Veith and Zimmerman 1967) and received the customary certificate. His formal medical education was not completed until 10 years after his apprenticeship, when he received a degree from the University of Pennsylvania, successor to the Medical College of Philadelphia.

Practicing only briefly after that, he assumed faculty positions at several fledgling medical schools, and became an energetic advocate for the expansion of academic education. An eloquent spokesman, he stated that licensed apprentices possessed only a "certificate of inferiority" (Kett 1968). Between his birth in 1795 and his death in 1852, the number of medical schools grew from 4 to 42 (Rothstein 1972). Unfortunately, lack of control of medical education allowed "diploma mills" to come into existence. Course fees charged directly by professors to enrolling students, tutorial fees and apprentice fees made it possible for faculty members at urban schools to earn as much as $10,000 annually when $1,000 per year was considered adequate income for a practicing physician (Rothstein 1972). With such inducements, it is no wonder that the number of medical colleges grew 10-fold in one lifespan. Without requirements, other than payment of fees, a student could receive an engraved diploma attesting to his qualifications to practice medicine.

## FRICTION CREATES REFORMS

Reform efforts, when they came, were the result of a schism between the medical educators and medical practitioners rather than the flagrant profiteering of some faculty. While envy was one source of friction, greed was another. Some of the more reputable and insightful medical schools added clinical practice sequences of instruction, which involved actual treatment of patients in a special dispensary designed for faculty—student use. This brought a flood of protest and resolution by the New York Academy of Medicine, which stated:

> *Whereas, the cliniques now held at the medical colleges as at present conducted, are or may be made tributary to the private interest of the professors at the expense of other and younger members of the profession, depriving them by an odious monopoly of practice and operation and often to fees to which they are justly entitled, therefore resolved, as the sense of this Academy, that to prescribe for or to operate upon the legitimate patients of any other physician, knowing them to be such, although done gratuitously at a clinique, is equally unwarrantable and unprofessional . . . and . . . is a violation of the code of medical ethics adopted by this body (Rothstein 1972).*

The schism was as damaging to the profession as were the substandard graduates of unregulated educational institutions. Medical societies were left with little control over the activities of the graduates because their diplomas were generally accepted in lieu of licensure. In Connecticut, medical society members were empowered to sit on the examining board of the Medical Institution of Yale College and could cast the deciding vote for or against graduation. However, this arrangement was the exception to the rule. For the most part, medical society activities were limited to heated condemnation (Rothstein 1972).

The substitution of diplomas for licensure also assumed dramatic proportions. New York, for example, licensed over 100 physicians in 1820, with 38 medical graduates exempted. By 1846, 246 graduates began to practice by virtue of a diploma alone, and only 10 licenses were issued. In the same year, the New York State Medical Society met to take a stand on medical education (Bordley and Harvey 1976). During its meeting, a resolution containing the following proposals was passed:

> *First. That it is expedient for the medical profession of the United States to institute a National Medical Association. Second. That it is desirable that a uniform and elevated standard of requirements for the degree of M.D. should be adopted by all the medical schools in the United States. Third. That it is desirable that young men, before being*

*received as students of medicine, should have acquired a suitable preliminary education. Fourth. That it is expedient that the medical profession in the United States should be governed by the same code of medical ethics.*

Another conference was called for the following year in Philadelphia, and during this second meeting the American Medical Association was founded. Its constitution was adopted with a preamble dedicating the organization's activities to advancement of medical knowledge, elevation of standards of education and ethics, and public information regarding the responsibilities and requirements of physicians (Veith 1967).

Concerted action did not take place as easily as had been expected, however. The schism between professor and practitioner continued within the newly formed organization. It was apparent that licensure mechanisms were, for all practical purposes, defunct. Reform of medical education did occur at the end of the nineteenth century, but it was not brought about by the medical profession. It was, rather, the result of academic movements instituted by a new breed of college presidents who had been educated in Europe, and who initiated a series of reforms designed to emulate European models (Bordley and Harvey 1976).

## TWENTIETH CENTURY AMERICA

By 1900, there were 160 medical schools in the United States, graduating an annual total of 5,600 students. Their curriculum was so poor, when compared to European universities, that an estimated 15,000 physicians traveled overseas to study medicine after finishing their American studies (Bowers and Purcell 1976).

Public apathy persisted during the first decade of the twentieth century in the face of inferior, and frequently dangerous, procedures. Unnecessary surgery was rampant, exacerbated by the custom of fee-splitting. Opium and alcohol were used indiscriminately, and with complete disregard for subsequent addiction. These abuses were created by the crowded medical market, with its depressing effect on the individual physician's income (Duffy 1976).

In 1903, after 30 irresolute years of internal debate, the American Medical Association finally took a tentative step toward reform with the creation of the Council on Medical Education. Its purpose was to study methods of improving medical education in the United States, although not necessarily to implement the recommendations.

In 1908, the Council on Medical Education, perceiving that an internal solution would not be forthcoming, sought an ally in the Carnegie Foundation (Bowers and Purcell 1976). At first they requested publication of their own report on medical school quality, but the Carnegie Foundation discarded the council's report and announced its intention to undertake its own survey. A chain of events that rapidly altered the character of medical education, practice, and organization was thus set in motion.

In 1910, under the innocuous title "Carnegie Foundation Bulletin No. Four," the foundation presented the findings of its survey. Its author, Abraham Flexner, remains dominantly associated with these findings today (Bowers and Purcell 1976):

1. 137 schools had nonexistent or unenforced entrance requirements.
2. 138 schools had teaching staffs composed entirely of physicians who maintained simultaneous independent practices.
3. Laboratory courses, where they existed, were poorly taught and inadequately equipped.
4. 140 schools had inadequate or nonexistent libraries.

The American press drew hungrily on the report, which shortly caused a major scandal. Diminished enrollment forced many schools to close their doors. By 1922, the quality of medical education had improved, but the flow in incoming professionals had been cut in half.

## AN INVESTIGATION OF HOSPITAL CONDITIONS

In 1912, the Clinical Congress of Surgeons, the first specialty branch in the American Medical Association, followed in the footsteps of the Council of Medical Education. Concerned about the conditions in American hospitals, which ranged from the inadequate to the filthy, they petitioned the Carnegie Foundation to undertake a study. The Carnegie Foundation concurred on the need for the project, but made a crucial change in method. Instead of conducting an impartial investigation of its own, it awarded funds directly to the Clinical Congress itself (Lembcke 1967). At the same time, an accrediting body for surgeons was formed within the Clinical Congress in 1913, calling itself the American College of Surgeons. This group stated as its purposes: elevation of the standard of surgery, establishment of standards of surgical competence, and the granting of fellowships to recognize surgeons with appropriate qualifications.

The outbreak of World War I forced a 4-year delay of the aforementioned study. Nevertheless, by 1920 the American College of Surgeons was able to develop a set of objective criteria against which to compare hospitals. In addition, these criteria were categorized to compare hospitals (Table 1).

Only this prototype survives, and the remainder of the survey has disappeared entirely. It is known that the survey began with larger hospitals, using a $75,000 additional grant from the Carnegie Foundation, and that preliminary findings indicated that only 89 of 692 hospitals studied met any reasonable standard whatsoever (Lembcke 1967). The

**Table 1.** One Hundred Cases of Chronic Appendicitis

| Procedures and Results | Number in Hospital 1 | Number in Hospital 2 |
|---|---|---|
| Complete physical examination including blood count | 100 | 14 |
| Number of consultations held | 41 | 2 |
| Working diagnoses recorded in advance of operation | 100 | None |
| Progress notes recorded by doctor | 100 | None |
| Infections following operation | 3 | 12 |
| Incorrect diagnoses | 4 | 14 |
| Number of patients relieved | 94 | 77 |
| Number of patients dead | 2 | 9 |

Note:   Reprinted with permission from Lembcke (1967).

procedures employed and the individual findings subsequently disappeared from the files of the college. Apparently, the survey committee ordered all records destroyed. The college subsequently announced a program,

> *first, to define a Minimum Standard; second, to enlist the cooperation of the hospitals in the fulfillment of the Standard, this work to be accomplished through personal visits to the hospitals by staff members of the College; and third, to publish from time to time the list of hospitals throughout the two countries which fulfilled the Minimum Standard (Lembcke 1967).*

Publication of the list would not take place until "the hospitals themselves generally approved of such publication, each hospital having been given full opportunity to meet the Standard under normal conditions."

The American College of Surgeons promoted this program for the next 30 years. Efforts were directed toward achieving uniformity in organization, staff discipline, supervision, review of records, regulation of practice, and adequacy of facilities and equipment (Lembcke 1967).

Long-range improvements were attempted through graduate training of specialists, organization of medical staff committees and hospital boards, and the promulgation of a set of Minimum Standards for Hospitals, for which a point-rating system was developed in 1948. These efforts continued until 1952, when the Joint Commission on the Accreditation of Hospitals was founded to perform these tasks. The standards were superficial and were not related directly to the quality of patient care, but only to the organization and function of the institution (Lembcke 1967).

A method for evaluating patient care had been developed well before World War I by Dr. E.A. Codman. Because of the institutional environment emphasis of the day, it lay dormant for 40 years. Called the "End Result System," Codman's program abstracted every case admitted from 1912 to 1916, classifying the outcome as "favorable" or "unfavorable with cause." Patients were also reevaluated after 1 year (Lembcke 1967).

The Joint Commission on the Accreditation of Hospitals revived interest in this method for evaluating patient care. They found that the program, called "Medical Audit," provided a means of discovering and addressing deficiencies in patient care. Medical Audit has been used since that time to supplement the structural certification of hospitals by the Joint Commission.

Specialty board certification, like that of the surgeon, had enjoyed the longest lifespan of any professionally dominated quality review program in the United States. The program was motivated by the unwillingness of most states to enforce certification as a precondition for specialty practice. To this day, physicians may establish practice in the specialty of choice after licensure. Hospitals, however, began to respect specialty board certification when selecting staff, thus providing economic incentives for participation to individual physicians.

## EMERGING GOVERNMENT ROLES

The most recent participant in the evolution of hospital-based quality assurance has been the United States government. Following passage of Title XVIII and XIX of the Social Security Act, demand for services by the newly insured aged and medically indigent increased so dramatically that a system of claims review was created by the Social Security Administration.

The mechanism called for establishment of utilization review committees, which would perform three functions: concurrent review, retrospective review, and retroactive denial of claims. The system was cumbersome, but it was put into action in hospitals across the country. After only a few years of operation, its deficiencies were apparent. Criteria for appropriateness had never been explicit, and the resulting confusion left utilization review committees in the center of a tug-of-war between the institution and physicians and their fiscal intermediary (Holloway and Wiczai 1974).

In 1969, the Senate Committee on Finance began a series of hearings that addressed the mounting public and private costs of medical care, chiefly with respect to Medicare and Medicaid. In these hearings, and subsequent communications with staff members, the concept of peer review was reintroduced. Hailed as a novel concept, it was, in fact, not untried. Twenty years earlier, physician groups in California had formed Foundations for Medical Care, which served both as referral sources for insurance coverage cases and as claims review mechanisms for those same patients. In California's San Joaquin Valley, peer review of patient care occurred as a routine part of the claims review process. A coordinating body, the United Foundations for Medical Care, began introducing this process into the activities of foundations in other areas of the country, and assisted in the design of alternative models for its operation.

The concept came to the attention of the Department of Health, Education and Welfare in the late 1960s, and grants were awarded to physician groups in several localities to establish Experimental Medical Care Review Organizations on a regional basis. Since these were physician-initiated, they met with more success than had been expected, especially in the state of Utah, which initiated a statewide structure.

In 1970, the American Medical Association, responding to a growing movement for a national health insurance program, introduced its own health insurance bill before Congress. The Fulton—Broyhill bill, also known as Medicredit, contained, among its other provisions, the stipulation that complaints regarding patient care be reviewed by peer review organizations (PROs) composed of physicians. The measure failed passage as a whole, but the PRO idea was not lost (Decker and Bonner 1973).

Late in 1969, Senator Wallace Bennett of Utah introduced the concept into the Social Security amendments as the Professional Standards Review Organization (PSRO). The amendments as a whole failed to clear the conference committee before the end of the 91st Congress, and were introduced in the 92nd Congress (Gasfield 1975).

On 30 October 1972, HR1 (House of Representatives Bill #1) became Public Law 92-603, a portion of which amended Article XI of the Social Security Act to include the establishment of PSROs. Local medical societies were given the option of designating themselves or their Foundation for Medical Care as PSROs, and an election system was designed to select among competing organizations to ensure the support of a majority of local physicians. Designated organizations were given provisional status and technical assistance in developing criteria for methods of assessing length of stay and adequacy of patient care. The Joint Commission for the Accreditation of Hospitals responded to this partial shift in function by assuming a new role in the development of optimal, diagnosis-specific criteria for patient care.

# THE LESSONS OF HISTORY

Society can regulate all practitioners of healing, whatever their persuasion, as demonstrated by the Faculty of Paris. It can regulate only medical practitioners, as did the Royal College; or certain specialties, as did the Chou Dynasty; or all followers of one school of thought, as did Hippocrates. Or society can certify only those who offer themselves for regulatory recognition, as was the case in Rome and twentieth-century America.

The needs of the health consumer and the needs of the healing professional do not necessarily coincide. Although regulation is ostensibly designed to protect the consumer from artful quackery, it can also, as we have seen among the Babylonians, prevent the consumer from receiving any health care whatsoever, except at a high price. Moreover, the consumer's view of quackery may not coincide with the mainstream professional's. The persons apprehended and tried by the Faculty of Paris had patients who defended the effectiveness of their treatment vigorously and openly. More recently, the homeopathic practitioners whom the Royal College sought to discredit have had wide followings, which exist to this day.

Sanctions brought to bear on health practitioners may be inducements to maintain or exceed a certain standard, or they may be deterrents against violating certain principles. As in the practice of medicine itself, the more stringent the sanctions are, the greater the potential for lasting damage. This was illustrated by centuries of blind adherence to Galen because of the church's power to institute devastating reprisal against dissenters. Public opinion, under competitive market conditions, both rewards and punishes, as Hippocrates realized. But regulatory actions also bring their actions, and reigns of terror deprived some societies of their best physicians.

Variations in standards appear to have been a function of two factors: (1) whether the standards were set by the profession itself or an external entity and (2) what level of proficiency they were designed to maintain. In the Hippocratic, profession-set form, standards consisted of a set of unacceptable behaviors, which formed a minimum below which it was inadvisable for the professional to fall. The Egyptians, on the other hand, transmitted all that they knew in medicine, in the expection that all professionals would strive toward this goal. Those societies that made use of academic credentials valued the existence of a norm held in common by the qualified.

## A CHOICE

The choice of standards is a crucial one. When coupled with stringency of enforcement, it frequently determined the rate at which professional knowledge grew or froze. Away from the oppressions of the Faculty of Paris, with its academic standards and its drastic reprisals, the profession developed. Elsewhere in France, it stultified.

Although manifestations of minimum, maximum, and normal standards appear in retrospect as happenstances rather than choices, in conscious planning situations they pose a dilemma. Does one set a minimum standard in the interest of practitioner availability, knowing that much second-rate conduct is bound to occur? Does one set the highest possible standards, sacrificing a pool of potentially adequate professionals? Is a norm an actual midpoint, or is it simply an agreed-on convenience? This debate has occurred throughout the centuries.

The healing process has at least three distinct stages that are potential areas for quality management: The physician (1) comes to the patient with a certain academic and experiential background; (2) treats the patient with a certain set of skills; and (3) leaves the patient with symptoms alleviated, worsened, or unchanged.

Assessment of quality can take place at any or all of these stages. It may be limited to examination of the credentials of the physician prior to beginning practice. The licensure efforts of the Caliph of Baghdad were addressed to this first stage, and in recent times such quality control activities have been defined as "structure"-related, indicating that the credentials are intended, or structured, to ensure quality of care. Assessment may be focused on the process of the healing act itself, as were the papyri of ancient Egypt. This dimension of quality assurance emphasizes and analyzes what occurs during treatment. Finally, assessment may occur after treatment, through a determination of whether treatment was effective or injurious. The Chinese of the Chou Dynasty chose the latter, counting, for simplicity's sake, the deaths that had occurred. Evaluation following care is now called outcome assessment, and it relies heavily on techniques that contrast the actual outcome, following treatment, to the expected prognosis.

In the final analysis, the lengthy history of medical quality assurance activities, including today's current techniques, must only be viewed as prologue to methodologies that may be developed in the future. The content and context of such future quality review programs is a challenge for all health care professionals.

## REFERENCES

Ackerknecht EH: A Short History of Medicine. New York, Ronald Press, 1955

Bell WJ Jr: The Colonial Physician and Other Essays. New York, Science History Publications, 1975

Bordley J III, Harvey AM: Two Centuries of American Medicine 1776–1976. Philadelphia, W. B. Saunders, 1976

Bowers JZ, Purcell EF: Advances in American Medicine: Essays at the Bicentennial. New York, Josiah Macy, Jr. Foundation, 1976

Cope Z: Sidelights on the History of Medicine. London, Butterworth and Co, 1957

Davis NS: History of Medicine with the Code of Medical Ethics. Chicago, Cleveland Press, 1903

Decker B, Bonner P: PSRO: Organization for Regional Peer Review. Cambridge, Mass, Ballinger Publishing Co, 1973

Duffy J: The Healers: The Rise of the Medical Establishment. New York, McGraw-Hill, 1976

Etziony MB: The Physician's Creed. Springfield, Ill, Charles C Thomas, 1973

Gordon MB: Aesculapius Comes to the Colonies. Ventnor, NJ, Centnor Publishers, 1949

Gosfield A: PSRO's: The Law and the Health Consumer. Cambridge, Mass, Ballinger Publishing Co, 1975

Holloway DC, Wiczai JL: PSRO's and the emerging role of hospital utilization review committees, in Occasional Papers in Hospital and Health Administration, No. 6. Berkeley, University of California School of Public Health, 1974

Kett JF: The Formation of the American Medical Profession. New Haven, Conn, Yale University Press, 1968

Kibre P: The faculty of medicine at Paris, charlatanism and unlicensed medical practices in the late Middle Ages. Bull Hist Med 27:1–20, 1953

Lembcke PA: Evolution of the Medical Audit. JAMA 199:111–118, 1967

McLachlan G, McKeown T (eds): Medical History and Medical Care: A Symposium of Perspectives. London, Oxford University Press, 1971

Nagel H: American Medicine. Translated by Sigerist HE. New York, W. W. Norton, 1934

Raach JH: A seventeenth century English medical license. Bull Hist Med 13:210–216, 1943

Rothstein WG: American Physicians in the Nineteenth Century. Baltimore, The Johns Hopkins University Press, 1972

Sigerist HE: Man and Medicine. New York, W. W. Norton, 1932

Sigerist HE: The history of medical licensure. JAMA 104: 1057–1060, 1935

Sigerist HE: Medicine and Human Welfare. New Haven, Conn, Yale University Press, 1941

Stenn F: The Growth of Medicine. Springfield, Ill, Charles C Thomas, 1967

Veith I: Government control and medicine in eleventh century China. Bull Hist Med 14:159–172, 1943

Veith I, Zimmerman LM: American Medicine 1607–1900. Chicago, Rand McNally, 1967

Venzmer G: Five Thousand Years of Medicine. New York, Taplinger, 1968

Wilcocks C: Medical Advance, Public Health and Social Evolution. Oxford, Pergammon Press, 1965

# 2

# A Brief History of the American Psychiatric Association's Involvement in Peer Review

*Gary L. Shepherd, M.D.*

# A Brief History of the American Psychiatric Association's Involvement in Peer Review

T hroughout history, peer review has helped to define the role and methods by which physicians practice. Medicine has likewise shaped the method, definition, and purpose of peer review. Thus peer review is as old as medicine and as new. This is true for all of medicine, including psychiatry.

Medicine cuts across all fields of science from sociology to physics. It is charged with evaluating, selecting, and integrating components from all the sciences that have an impact on the prevention, evaluation, and treatment of ill health or the maintenance of good health. If medicine's only charge was the application of scientific principles, it would need only technicians, not physicians. However, medicine has another charge: to interact with people intimately. It must consider their emotions (which are not always rational), their perceptions (which can often be distorted to a greater or lesser degree), and their ability to communicate (which often is impaired by their perception and their emotions). Furthermore, medical care is affected by the ability to understand and cooperate—a function of all of the above.

A useful oversimplification follows. We ask: How do you feel? Where does it hurt? Can you describe the pain? Is it worse at one time than at another? Why did you stop taking the medication?

We say: If you will take one of these t.i.d. you will feel much better. Just follow this diet and those symptoms will go away. It is very important that you try to relax; getting upset doesn't really help anything and it makes your blood pressure go up.

We lament: If she had only followed my advice, surgery would not have been necessary. If he would only stay on his medication, these hospitalizations would not be necessary. If he could have communicated that distress to me, I might have been able to help prevent his suicide.

By acknowledging these vicissitudes of humanity, we are transformed from technicians to physicians. This is the art of medicine—combining the requisite skills of a technician to treat symptomatology with insights into the patients' feelings and perceptions. It is clear why sound clinical judgment is a cornerstone of medicine and a hallmark of the good physician. Furthermore, it verifies that psychiatry's roots are found within medicine.

Peer review actually provides a significant educational process for the medical student. Rounds, grand rounds, and supervision test not only the students' technical skills, but their ability to interact with both patients and staff effectively. The physician in training finishes the basic science portion of the training fairly quickly. From that time forward, most of the training is done in the context of peer review-like activities. First, the "student physician" will receive input and guidance from those in the student's chosen field who are one to one hundred or more steps ahead. In my junior year of medical school, my classmates and I were taught by senior medical students, interns, residents, clinical faculty, and professors of medicine. We also helped each other. With each step forward (the more senior we became), the amount of input and ideas from those at our own level increased. Now, as a member of the senior clinical staff of a teaching facility, I enjoy the exchanges that take place in grand rounds, in staffing patients, and in individual supervision. The major differences among those of us involved in these activities is the amount of experience. Sometimes I teach, sometimes I learn.

After completion of formal training, physicians are eligible to obtain a license to practice and to obtain staff privileges at various hospitals. Recommendations from peers is of major importance in these determinations. They may also wish to receive board certification or to apply for fellowships. In these instances, another form of peer review—face-to-face review by other psychiatrists—is required.

The practice of medicine and psychiatry as a specialty of medicine has largely been defined through peer review. Peer review often leads to the development of criteria and guidelines that help us define such things as "usual and customary," "medical necessity," "appropriate care" for a diagnosis, and the ethics of our profession. In view of all this, it is not surprising that when third-party payers wanted to set severe and arbitrary limits on psychiatric coverage, the profession quickly advocated the use of peer review as opposed to arbitrary limits.

With the foregoing as a background, let us now look at the recent history of peer review as it relates to third-party payers and psychiatry. Current peer review of psychiatric services has its origins at both the district branch level and at the national level through components of the American Psychiatric Association (APA). National peer review activities have received oversight, input, and direction from governing bodies, from APA's board, assembly, councils, and Committee on Peer Review, and from many of the district branches themselves. Psychiatric peer review activities came into being soon after third-party payers began to provide benefits for mental disorders.

An important distinction should be made at this point. When I speak of peer review, I am talking about those peer review activities that were developed within our profession. I am not talking about the activities of Professional Standards Review Organizations (PSROs); PSROs were primarily the result of the governmental regulatory process with limited professional input allowed.The former represents a major effort initiated by mainstream psychiatry through the APA and its district branches. The latter does not.

I would also like to make it clear at the beginning that the history I intend to provide in this chapter is simply an overview. It will be an historical perspective from which to view the chapters that are to follow. To chronicle completely the history of psychiatric peer review since 1970 and the people who were responsible would require a book in itself. I hope someday this will be done. Naturally, if one does not present the entire history, one presents a more biased history. My bias will be based on an increasingly intense and personal involvement with peer review and peer review concepts and processes. It began in 1971 in the San Diego district branch and then the California Psychiatric Association. It led me to become involved in much of what has been developed on a national level through my participation on the APA Peer Review Committee and the APA's National Advisory Council to the Civilian Health and Medical Program of the Uniformed Services (CHAMPUS).

In 1966, Congress directed CHAMPUS to include inpatient and outpatient psychiatric treatment in their benefits package. At about the same time, the Federal Employees Health Benefits Program (FEHBP) added similar benefits.

The private insurance sector also began providing psychiatric benefits that were generally more restrictive than those offered by CHAMPUS or the FEHBP. Those plans that did provide coverage by mental illnesses limited the number of inpatient days or outpatient visits and set high deductibles or low lifetime maximums. Originally, they also attempted to limit coverage to services provided by physicians.

The introduction of mental health benefits occurred prior to the establishment of guidelines regarding the diagnosis or treatment of mental illness. There was no consensus regarding reasonable utilization of services or the appropriateness of care for given dysfunctions. As a result, third-party payers needed assistance in making benefit decisions, particularly in regions with high utilization rates of mental health services. The formation of insurance and peer review committees within the district branches in the late 1960s and into the 1970s represented an attempt by organized psychiatry to offer third-party payers its technical expertise. In some areas, our help was accepted; in others, these attempts were met with suspicion and resistance. In yet other instances, third-party payers sought the help of psychiatry but received little cooperation. In a few instances, there was outright resistance.

The APA was also aware of these evolving concerns. Consequently, as peer review activities increased at the district branch level, they began developing at the national level as well. The Office of CHAMPUS (OCHAMPUS) gradually became aware of the APA's ability and willingness to provide help and expertise in the areas of utilization and quality assurance. This led to cooperative efforts between OCHAMPUS and the APA. This cooperation and involvement was the foundation from which peer review as an alternative to arbitrary limits on psychiatric benefits by third-party payers was developed on a national level.

The private practice of psychiatry would have been on the decline had psychiatry not taken the initiative to work with public and private health insurance forces. Individual psychiatrists convinced district branches to develop peer review concepts and methods, which, in turn, influenced our national association. In fact, many of those individual psychiatrists gave a significant amount of time and energy to develop and work on APA committees in addition to working for their district branches. They felt that peer review needed to be a statement of organized psychiatry rather than just of individual psychiatrists.

As stated above, Congress amended existing legislation in 1966 and enabled CHAMPUS to provide payment for psychiatric care in addition to already authorized obstetrical, surgical, and general medical care. Under CHAMPUS' psychiatric coverage, there were no limitations. In effect, Congress gave the CHAMPUS program a blank check to pay for this expansion of its benefits package. In addition, there was no method for evaluating the medical necessity or appropriateness of care.

In 1967, psychiatric costs for CHAMPUS were $8.8 million—about 7 percent of the budget. By 1973, psychiatric costs had grown to almost $92 million—about 22 percent of the budget (Office of the Civilian Health and Medical Program 1977).

CHAMPUS philosophy with regard to utilization review and quality assurance had not changed from that of the early military medicare period (1956–1966) to 1973. During that time, CHAMPUS contracted with private insurance companies to process claims for services rendered by the civilian medical community. Blue Cross/Blue Shield Plans and Mutual of Omaha were the primary fiscal administrators. In some states, medical associations also paid CHAMPUS claims.

The administrators in OCHAMPUS' Denver office were anxious for the medical community to accept its military medicare program in its early years. This was accomplished by avoiding conflict about payment and eligibility. This attitude did not change until 1974, when OCHAMPUS bowed to the expertise of insurance companies who were experienced in paying doctors and hospital claims. As a result, OCHAMPUS turned to the established indemnity plans for utilization review of claims because they were already respected by the civilian medical community.

The broader benefit package, which went into effect in early 1967, caused a great deal of turmoil for the traditional insurance companies. They had never dealt with the type of claims that began to rush in from CHAMPUS beneficiaries. Many benefits that had traditionally been considered too risky by commercial insurance carriers were now included in the CHAMPUS benefits package. Payment of those claims were often delayed in late 1967 when inquiries from insurance companies to the CHAMPUS office regarding when, how, and to whom payment should be made went unanswered.

A Case Review Committee (CRC), which began to evaluate and interpret the new benefits package, was formed within OCHAMPUS. The committee functioned from 1967 through 1971. Its decisions (essentially payment policy for CHAMPUS) were sometimes inconsistent. Review of the CRC's minutes demonstrates a distinct association between interpretations of benefits available and the committee member's backgrounds. When physicians dominated the CRC, benefit decisions were conservative. When nonphysicians dominated, benefit decisions were very liberal. Throughout that period, the management philosophy of CHAMPUS continued to support the concept that the major insurance companies had the most expertise and capability for reviewing questionable cases and providing third-level (professional) review when required.

OCHAMPUS set no limits on hospital charges until 1974. Prior to that time, there was wide disparity in hospital expenses, with room and board charges ranging from $700 a month to over $3,000 a month. OCHAMPUS did not negotiate charges with hospitals and did not require any financial data to justify the rates charged.

In keeping with the philosophy described above, OCHAMPUS did not pay claims directly. Instead, it delegated this authority to approximately 45 fiscal agents, primarily Blue Cross/Blue Shield plans and Mutual of Omaha. This is how a claim was paid: A person who needed psychiatric care selected a hospital from a list of approved CHAMPUS hospitals. No audit or spot check was ever made to determine whether CHAMPUS claimants were actually eligible. Once a patient was hospitalized, the sponsor signed a blank CHAMPUS claim form. At the end of the month, the hospital completed this form by listing the charges accumulated that month. The claim form was then submitted to the appropriate fiscal agent. Each of the fiscal agents periodically sent a bill listing what had been paid out for CHAMPUS beneficiaries to the CHAMPUS office and was reimbursed.

The fiscal agents processing the claims for CHAMPUS performed desk audits of the claims. No provision was made for on-site audits or even spot checks to verify whether the claims were being submitted for eligible persons, the accuracy of admission and discharges, the dates therapy was actually given, or that medications were actually administered.

In addition to poor auditing procedures, CHAMPUS had no accreditation requirements or site review procedures. Instead, it relied on state and local licensing laws and authorities to deal with unsavory institutions. Unfortunately this rarely occurred. More than 1,000 individual institutions were approved by OCHAMPUS to provide long-term (over 90 days) psychiatric treatment (U.S. Senate 1974). Most of these organizations receiving OCHAMPUS approval were legitimate. However, it was possible for a private school that had been denied accreditation as a school by state authorities to apply for and receive approval by CHAMPUS as a psychiatric hospital if a psychiatrist visited it at periodic intervals.

As a result, a large portion of CHAMPUS money reimbursed adolescent psychiatric care. Because of poor record keeping, CHAMPUS was unable to specify the number of such facilities treating its beneficiaries. However, privately owned, commercial "psychiatric hospitals" or "residential psychiatric treatment centers" sprang up all over the country. Juvenile authorities at the state, county, and local levels discovered that it was more convenient for them to subcontract the care of troubled adolescents to such commercial institutions (frequently in far-removed states) than it was to find a foster home or other appropriate placement nearby. These institutions, also known as "commercially operated jails," were eager to obtain CHAMPUS patients because there was no limit on what they could charge.

In 1972, in an attempt to bring the fiscal administration of CHAMPUS under control, the assistant secretary of defense (health affairs) was delegated oversight responsibility for the administration of CHAMPUS benefits. This had previously been the responsibility of the surgeon general of the army. Immediately an overall review of CHAMPUS coverage and operations was begun (Asher 1981).

Program operation changes ensued. Some of the changes involved revisions of earlier management control efforts by the Department of Defense (DOD). For example, approval for inpatient psychiatric care beyond 45 days was granted by a central review department if it was determined that the care documented in the patient's treatment plan could not be more effectively or economically provided elsewhere. This review department was directed by a military physician and staffed by professional social work personnel who understood the availability and types of mental health services. However, the DOD discontinued this system in 1974, citing its failure to be cost effective.

In February 1973, Kenneth Wooden, Executive Director of the Institute of Applied Politics, Princeton, New Jersey, published a study describing the state of Illinois' residential treatment centers (Wooden 1976). Adolescents living at these centers and in need of psychiatric care were treated like inmates at state detention centers. By court order, children were shipped across state lines to obtain "treatment." This was particularly true if the children were beneficiaries of CHAMPUS. Mr. Wooden visited OCHAMPUS in late 1973 and talked with members of the staff. Through a series of conversations, he learned of CHAMPUS involvement in residential treatment centers.

In 1973 there were 3,000 children in 540 residential treatment centers across the country (Wooden 1976). There were no national standards for such centers. OCHAMPUS' attempts to withdraw funding from many of these institutions resulted in litigation. In many instances the courts ruled in favor of the institutions while at the same time hundreds of children continued to suffer abuse and were denied treatment in this very large profit-making industry.

Several pressures were converging on CHAMPUS at the same time; the DOD was experiencing severe funding problems due to Vietnam and the Office of Management and Budget was pressuring CHAMPUS to control its expenditures. This led the assistant secretary of defense (health affairs) to make major changes in CHAMPUS policies during the 1975 budget cycle. He required that all inpatient treatment facilities obtain accreditation from the Joint Commission on Accreditation of Hospitals as a condition for CHAMPUS reimbursement. This policy reduced the number of institutions that were eligible for CHAMPUS payments from over 1,000 to 485. (Asher 1981). Unfortunately, the assistant secretary also made a number of drastic, arbitrary cuts in the psychiatric benefit. For example, beneficiaries were allowed only 120 inpatient days per year and the number of outpatient sessions was limited to 40 visits per year.

The severe curtailing of CHAMPUS benefits created significant problems for the large majority of CHAMPUS beneficiaries as well as for the providers of care. This attempt to "throw out the baby with the bath water" was not left unchallenged. The American Psychiatric Association galvanized itself into action. In late 1974 and early 1975, the curtailment of benefits was formally protested by the APA to the secretary of defense and the House and Senate committees appropriating and authorizing OCHAMPUS' budget. In addition to its concern, the APA also made it clear that it had the interest and the expertise to help.

At about the same time as the fiscal crisis was developing, the Senate Permanent Subcommittee on Investigations began its CHAMPUS hearings. The four-day hearings, beginning on 23 July 1974, concentrated on adolescent psychiatric care in OCHAMPUS-approved institutions (U.S. Senate 1974). The investigation was fueled by a series of critical General Accounting Office reports. Faced with an apparent scandal involving several residential treatment centers, OCHAMPUS lacked the basic demographic information about its residential treatment center beneficiaries, as well as the technical expertise to manage this problem. They were clearly in need of help.

The APA's presence was not accidental. I have indicated earlier that organized psychiatry at the district branch and national level in the early 1970s was already developing guidelines and criteria to help ensure quality and manage costs. Because psychiatry was willing and able to do this as an organization, it carried more impact and higher visibility. Thus, even at that point, the APA recognized that organized psychiatry must advocate high-quality mental health services. To do this, standards were needed.

In 1971, the APA assembled a Task Force on Peer Review and Standards. Members from the APA's seven area divisions participated. The task force's mission was to develop PSRO standards and criteria; PSROs were in their infancy. The first model criteria sets (American Psychiatric Association 1973) were forerunners to the APA's *Manual of Psychiatric Peer Review* (American Psychiatric Association 1976). The model criteria sets were well received, and psychiatry had the distinction of being the first medical specialty to produce PSRO standards. Sadly, the PSRO movement never utilized organized psychiatry in the way and to the degree hoped. However, the APA benefited from that experience and at the same time utilization review and quality assurance were elevated on both the local and national fronts.

It is important to note that then and since, the central office and officers of the APA have viewed the development of peer review activities in what Donald Hammersley, M.D., APA Deputy Medical Director, has called a binary system approach (personal communication). This means that local branches have been encouraged to provide peer review services to the maximum degree possible. Many district branches have established programs in conjunction with local or regional insurance plans. The APA provided assistance, whenever possible, and limited its efforts to national plans whose coverage includes beneficiaries from several states.

To facilitate this exchange of information between members (also referred to as the binary system concept), the APA appointed Richard Dorsey, M.D., to act as its Field Consultant in Peer Review in the spring of 1976. He provided on-site information and guidance to all interested district branches to help them develop local Peer Review Committees.

The Task Force on Peer Review, first chaired by Frank Sullivan, was later named the Commission on Standards of Practice and Third Party Payers. The APA used the commission to voice its concerns to Congress and also provided technical assistance by offering to share its model criteria sets as industry guidelines. As a result, the findings of the Senate committee were influenced by the APA's participation.

On Thursday, 25 July 1974, Senator Jackson concluded the investigation into the CHAMPUS scandal with the following remarks:

> As to the CHAMPUS program itself . . . the objectives of the CHAMPUS program and, specifically, the psychiatric care of children, are laudatory. After hearing the testimony of the past few days, I feel even more convinced that the program must be put in order and administered so that its beneficiaries can fully benefit from Federal tax dollars. But words alone will not solve our problems. Nor will unilateral cutbacks by the Defense Department as was recently announced with regard to psychiatric care. We must take affirmative action. I am today calling upon the Department of Defense to submit to the Subcommittee—within thirty days—proposed regulations or administrative orders or amendments to the CHAMPUS Act which will establish controls and accountability for all CHAMPUS funding of institutions which we have studied at our hearing (U.S. Senate 1974).

This led to the formation of the now famous Select Committee on Psychiatric Care and Evaluation (SCOPCE). It was formed by the National Institute of Mental Health (NIMH) with the aid of the APA, and funded by the DOD.

The initial conference to discuss SCOPCE's goals was held in Washington, D.C., in November 1974. All 65 persons invited to participate at the meeting attended, exceeding the hopes of Dane G. Prugh, M.D., Chairman of the SCOPCE Committee. At the conference, Mr. Vernon McKenzie, Principal Deputy Assistant Secretary of Defense (Health Affairs), spoke of the importance of the project initiated by the DOD and the NIMH. In October of 1974, the SCOPCE committee began the difficult task of developing a model program to monitor the treatment of children living in residential treatment centers.

At the first SCOPCE meeting, 16 interdisciplinary teams were formed. Each had a psychiatrist and a member of one or two other related mental health disciplines (psychology, social work, or nursing). This initial phase was based on the review of written material pertaining to diagnostic evaluation, treatment planning, and outcome measures. The teams reviewed more than 1,000 cases by July 1975.

In general, SCOPCE reviews (Select Committee on Psychiatric Care and Evaluation 1974) were conducted as follows: Prior to or on the 120th day of hospitalization, a summary of clinical documentation was sent to OCHAMPUS. It was then screened by first- and second-level reviewers using criteria provided by SCOPCE. The review criteria consisted of six administrative and seven treatment criteria, any one of which would lead to a third-level (professional) review. Administrative criteria triggering peer review included all cases in which:

a. Costs above the basic monthly charge exceeded $220 a month.
b. The base costs were greater than $60 a day, $1,800 a month, or $21,000 a year.
c. The patient was in the residence for more than 2 years.
d. There were more than three admissions to the same facility within 1 year.
e. There were more than three different facility admissions in 1 year.
f. There was an indication that paramedical personnel were being used for guarding or prohibiting a suicide.

The seven treatment criteria that initiated third-level review were cases in which:

a. Individual therapy was given by a psychiatrist more than three times a week.
b. There was an indication of psychoanalysis.
c. Shock treatment was administered.
d. There were more than two types of therapy per week.
e. The patient was receiving more than three psychotropics per day.
f. The patient received megavitamin therapy.

If a case demonstrated any one of the above criteria, it was sent to one of 16 review teams for consideration before benefits were continued.

After review by a multidisciplinary team, the case was sent back to CHAMPUS using forms developed by the NIMH. The recommendation was not restricted to a pay/no pay decision. Instead, the teams commented on the appropriateness of the patient's setting and treatment. Further care was often recommended in a different program.

Although the majority of disturbed children and adolescents were placed in appropriate residential treatment centers, a significant number were found to have been inappropriately placed and many had reached the point of maximum benefit from such a placement. Thus a savings of an estimated $5 million to CHAMPUS was made possible (Sorenson J: Report on Cost Savings of SCOPCE I. Unpublished report performed under NIMH contract. Rockville, Maryland, NIMH, 1975).

SCOPCE produced admission guidelines and continuing stay criteria based on medical necessity and clinical judgment by which CHAMPUS could begin to evaluate care rendered in residential treatment centers. These guidelines were in great part responsible for OCHAMPUS rescinding the cuts previously made in inpatient and outpatient mental health care. In addition, CHAMPUS was beginning to realize that there was an ally in the APA. They were now listening (although not fully convinced) to the APA's assertions that costs could be controlled and that the quality of care improved by means of peer review. Thus peer review was advocated as an alternative to arbitrary limits.

During the period between the formation of SCOPCE I and a follow-up project that became known as SCOPCE II, the APA continued to develop standards and criteria regarding the practice of psychiatry. In 1975, the APA Committee on Peer Review became a standing committee of the newly formed Commission on Standards of Practice and Third Party Payers. Dr. Donald G. Langsley was its first chair. One of the committee's primary tasks was to develop the *Manual of Psychiatric Peer Review* (American Psychiatric Association 1976). The manual addresses different treatment populations and modalities. For example, the American Academy of Child Psychiatry developed model criteria sets concerning the psychiatric treatment of children and adolescents. In addition, the American Psychoanalytic Association developed a section on diagnostic criteria for analyzability. There was also a general section that addressed many of the other issues dealing with the vicissitudes of peer review, such as advocacy, ethics, educational aspects, and confidentiality.

The *Manual of Psychiatric Peer Review* (American Psychiatric Association 1976) is a unique document. As previously stated, psychiatry was among the first medical specialty groups to develop peer review methods and standards for care. No other specialty group had such a complete document and, in fact, this document served as a major sourcebook for other developing peer review programs. Furthermore, it gave psychiatry a level of accountability and credibility it had not previously enjoyed. Soon after the publication of the first edition, work began on a revised version that would be even more complete (American Psychiatric Association 1981). This manual was used as a sourcebook in the development of the SCOPCE II project in San Diego.

SCOPCE II, supported by DOD and NIMH, came into being as a result of the success of SCOPCE I in 1975. It focused on the hospital treatment of adult schizophrenics because more CHAMPUS inpatient dollars went toward the treatment of patients with this diagnosis than for any other psychiatric diagnosis. SCOPCE II was implemented at the local level. For example, the Virginia Area V PSRO affiliated with the Colonial Medical Foundation in Norfolk, Virginia, conducted one study. The Norfolk area had been identified as one of the highest CHAMPUS utilization areas in the United States. Another project was administered in San Diego County in Southern California. That contract involved NIMH/DOD (OCHAMPUS), the APA district branch, and the San Diego Psychiatric Society (SDPS). Because of an extremely large CHAMPUS population, it helped to pioneer the development of peer review concepts and capabilities in the mid-1970s.

During the negotiation period of the San Diego project, several representatives of OCHAMPUS made it clear that they still had doubts about peer review. Some within OCHAMPUS predicted that the San Diego project would demonstrate our inability to be cost effective. Many felt it was like "letting the fox watch the chickens." If it failed, they could make a strong case for OCHAMPUS placing arbitrary limits on psychiatric care as had been done in 1974. With these pressures, the "San Diego experience" began.

For the project to work, it had to have the acceptance of the membership of the SDPS. That required a high level of communication with and education of the membership. Most of it took place in face-to-face meetings. Presentations were delivered and question-and-answer sessions were conducted at many monthly scientific meetings. I attended staff meetings at several psychiatric hospitals. Mailings described in detail how the project would operate. After initial suspicion, the membership soon realized that the project was not a police action but an opportunity to prove that ongoing professional review could work. The SDPS began to value the review process and was pleased that the system utilized peers from the same geographic area. We wished to show that we could review ourselves and, by doing so, could not only contain costs but improve the quality of services.

It was interesting to see that reviewing psychiatrists tended to be hard-nosed evaluators. There was no "rubber stamp" problem. In fact, it came to our attention that some reviewers were overly critical, thus requiring supervisory contacts with them to review these findings.

From the profession's point of view and that of OCHAMPUS, the project went well. OCHAMPUS was impressed with its organization and function. They were also pleased that SDPS was able to meet their needs in a very professional and effective manner.

Before SCOPCE II was over, OCHAMPUS and the DOD wanted to contract with the SDPS to expand the concurrent review program to cover all psychiatric admissions in San Diego County. The expanded program would include children and adolescents as well as adults. A proposal was developed for OCHAMPUS during SCOPCE II; in July 1977, we started a new contract for the concurrent review of *all* psychiatric diagnoses admitted to hospitals in San Diego County.

Oversight of these two contracts was led by OCHAMPUS, John Meyers, M.D., Lt. Cmdr., M.C., USA. Dr. Meyers became very interested in peer review as a result of the San Diego project. He convinced DOD to consider a third SCOPCE project to develop national criteria for all OCHAMPUS beneficiaries treated for mental disorders.

In late 1976 and early 1977, Dr. Meyers and OCHAMPUS entered into negotiations with the APA regarding a national review program. Donald Hammersley, M.D., the negotiator for the APA, helped bring about a contract between OCHAMPUS and the APA. The contract was signed in July 1977 and led to the formation of the APA's National Advisory Committee (NAC) to OCHAMPUS. Its task was to develop a national peer review system for inpatient and outpatient psychiatric treatment.

The first chair of the APA's NAC was Henry Altman, M.D. APA members from around the country with expertise and experience in peer review activities were invited to be members of the committee. The NAC was composed of psychoanalysts, child psychiatrists, medical directors of large hospitals, professors, and general practitioners in private practice—all of whom brought their enthusiasm and experience. Actually, if the committee members had fully understood the burden of work and the untold hours that the work would require, they might have reconsidered participating. Even after 5 years, I am still awed by the enormity of the task that the NAC and the APA undertook.

The APA hired Norman Penner to become the executive director of its Office of Peer Review. Mr. Penner has a master's degree in Public Health Administration. Prior to becoming executive director, he was special assistant to the assistant secretary of defense (health affairs) for CHAMPUS policy. He had participated in the SCOPCE projects as well as supervised the writing of the first comprehensive description of the CHAMPUS benefits package, and codified the programs' operations into the DOD's CHAMPUS regulation.

The committee began working in September 1977. It met three to four times a year thereafter. A first working draft of the peer review protocol was completed in 6 months. However, serious negotiations occurred for almost a year because OCHAMPUS' cost-cutting priorities conflicted with the APA's quality-control system. The NAC refused, however, to yield to pressures to produce a list of deniable benefits. Eventually in late 1978, key personnel changes in Denver resulted in a better working relationship between the APA and OCHAMPUS. This permited the NAC to proceed with its work in developing written procedures and criteria for peer review.

Not surprisingly, such a comprehensive and far-reaching peer review document caused considerable debate within the APA. For example, serious questions and concerns regarding confidentiality were raised. In addition, there were those who simply did not like the idea of being reviewed. Some district branches felt that a national program might interfere with their own locally developed relationships with third-party payers. Others saw peer review as a police force seeking to destroy psychiatry. There were even those who felt that the proposed peer review system did not go far enough in "policing" psychiatry and called it a whitewash. In fact, in 1976 (in the midst of San Diego's very successful and well-received SCOPCE II program), I had a visit from a colleague who accused me of being a "Judas goat" leading psychiatry down the road to ruin. It is evident that peer review provokes a wide variety of opinions and great emotion within the membership of the APA.

The NAC wanted to be certain that the new CHAMPUS peer review system was agreeable to the majority of APA members. Presentations during APA assembly and board of trustees meetings enabled divergent issues to be addressed. In addition, proposed procedures and screening criteria were sent to each district branch for evaluation and comment on two different occasions. This was followed by personal appearances by Norman Penner and members of the NAC at district branches and area councils to explain the intent and operations of the APA/CHAMPUS contract. The public discussions not only allayed some of the fears and concerns of the membership, but also helped produced acceptable screening criteria and instructions for CHAMPUS claims processors for administering the CHAMPUS' mental health peer review program. The instructions and screening criteria eventually became the CHAMPUS manual (Office of Civilian Health and Medical Program of the Uniformed Services 1980).

The purpose of the manual was to provide assistance to CHAMPUS claims processors (insurance companies) in selecting treatment episodes that would benefit from professional review. Thus screening criteria were not developed as rigid standards. Instead, they sought to identify certain cases that demonstrated utilization of diagnostic or treatment methods not commonly employed by most practicing psychiatrists.

The peer review system required the recruitment and appointment of peer reviewers nationally. Peer reviewers were nominated by their district branches. The district branches were asked to select psychiatrists who would reflect expertise and experience in adult general psychiatry, child and adolescent psychiatry, and psychoanalysis. These were the three divisions formally recognized in the APA's *Manual of Psychiatric Peer Review* (American Psychiatric Association 1976). Eventually a roster of over 400 psychiatrists across the nation was compiled.

While the APA/CHAMPUS project was being established, major developments were occuring in other areas as well. By late 1979, the Medical Directors' Committee of the Health Insurance Association of America was recommending the APA's model of peer review to other medical specialties. With reviewers in place and the manual in print, the APA's program was considered a model for the entire private insurance industry. This resulted in more work for the APA's Committee on Peer Review.

In 1979, that committee was already very busy with an expansion and revision of the manual. The new edition added several new sections relating to concurrent review of psychoanalysis, the evaluation of long-term hospital care, the use of electroconvulsive therapy, and model psychopharmacologic screening criteria. Furthermore, the model criteria sets were changed to reflect the revised diagnostic criteria contained within the *Diagnostic and Statistical Manual of Mental Disorders* (American Psychiatric Association 1980).

William Guillette, M.D., then medical director of Aetna Life and Casualty, was very enthusiastic about what psychiatry had to offer. When Aetna entered into a peer review agreement with the APA in August of 1979, this was only the beginning. As this historical overview is being written, 30 or more additional private insurance companies have entered into similar contracts with the APA.

In San Diego during this period, the concurrent review program described earlier continued. Because of its ongoing success, OCHAMPUS asked the SDPS to do an additional project also dealing with residential treatment facilities for children and adolescents. SDPS was asked to write a state-of-the-art paper concerning quality care in residential treatment centers. Additionally, guidelines and criteria were to be developed to evaluate the appropriateness and medical necessity of admissions and continued care. This led to a model program for review of residential treatment center care in San Diego County involving three facilities. Later, when DOD considered imposing arbitrary cuts on this benefit, OCHAMPUS and others pointed to the San Diego project as offering a more reasonable alternative that was cost effective and assured the quality of care. The San Diego residential treatment center review project served as a basis for the development of a national review program for residential treatment centers. OCHAMPUS requested that this program be conducted by the APA's Office of Peer Review.

The APA CHAMPUS Peer Review project became fully operational in January 1980. The results to date indicate that it has been effective in reducing costs without decreasing medically necessary care.

The San Diego project ended in January 1983, and now OCHAMPUS has contracted with the SDPS to do some valuable research of the data collected.

The APA-CHAMPUS National Advisory Committee continued to refine CHAMPUS peer review procedures and screening criteria. In addition, it participated in several special projects for CHAMPUS such as helping to establish criteria, guidelines, and standards for partial hospitalization and day treatment programs. Hopefully, these efforts will result in OCHAMPUS eventually including day treatment programs as a benefit. Again, CHAMPUS has used the peer review format to control costs and to ensure that mental health services are medically necessary and of good quality.

Peer review in American psychiatry has come of age. One by-product is that psychiatry's image has vastly improved. Our profession has credibility and accountability because we have "put our house in order." Peer review is important to the continued acceptance and growth of psychiatry.

Through district branches and our central office, the APA continues to break new ground. However, much more needs to be done. Peer review as developed by the APA is not static but a living, evolving system.

## REFERENCES

American Psychiatric Association: Model Criteria Sets. (Developed by the Ad Hoc Committee on PSROs.) Washington, DC, American Psychiatric Association, 1973

American Psychiatric Association: Manual of Psychiatric Peer Review, 1st ed. Washington, DC, American Psychiatric Association, 1976

American Psychiatric Association: Diagnostic and Statistical Manual of Mental Disorders, 3rd ed. Washington, DC, American Psychiatric Association, 1980

American Psychiatric Association: Manual of Psychiatric Peer Review, 2nd ed. Washington, DC, American Psychiatric Association, 1981

Asher J: Assuring Quality Mental Health Services: The CHAMPUS Experience (DHHS Publication No. ADM 81-1099). Rockville, Maryland; Alcohol, Drug Abuse, and Mental Health Administration, 1981

Office of Civilian Health and Medical Program of the Uniformed Services: CHAMPUS Chartbook, 1st ed. Aurora, Colorado; Office of Program Analysis and Statistics Division, 1977

Office of Civilian Health and Medical Program of the Uniformed Services: Manual for Inpatient and Outpatient Psychiatric Claims Review. Aurora, Colorado, Office of Civilian Health and Medical Program of the Uniformed Services, 1980

Select Committee on Psychiatric Care and Evaluation (SCOPCE): Minutes and files. Provided by Norman R. Penner, Lt. Col., U.S.A.F., MSC (Ret). 61, 1974

Wooden K: Weeping in the Playtime of Others: America's Incarcerated Children. New York, McGraw-Hill, 1976

U.S. Senate, 93rd Congress: Defense Departments' CHAMPUS Program (hearings before the Permanent Subcommittee on Investigations of the Committee on Government Operations, Parts 1 and 2, 23–26 July 1974). Washington, DC, U.S. Government Printing Office, 1974

# 3

# Ethical and Legal Aspects of Peer Review

*George F. Wilson, M.D.*

# Ethical and Legal Aspects
# of Peer Review

*Medicine is not a science, but a learned profession deeply rooted in a number of sciences, and charged with the obligation to apply them for man's benefit. Traditionally, this applying is made with compassion and in accord with a widely recognized moral and ethical code. Thus the responsibilities of medicine: to generate scientific knowledge and teach it to others, to use the knowledge for the health of an individual or a whole community, and to judge the moral and ethical propriety of each medical act that directly affects another human being (Cecil 1971).*

This quotation from the opening page of the *Cecil-Loeb Textbook of Medicine* provides a succinct summary of the basic principles of medical ethics, and is a useful starting point for examining the ethical issues

raised by the peer review process. Two obligations are described that are most relevant to our discussion: (1) the
responsibility to attend to the health of the entire community as well as the individual patient and (2) the moral
obligation to judge the propriety of each act of medical care
that comes to our attention. These two obligations, which
are incumbent on each individual physician as well as on
the profession as a whole, together point out the essential
tension between the responsibility to an individual patient
and the responsibility to the community of patients and
potential patients. This tension underlies many of the basic
issues in psychiatric ethics. This chapter will outline how
these ethical issues apply to psychiatric peer review and
how these ethical problems have led to the development of
legal restraints and protections for the peer review process.

## ETHICAL DIMENSIONS OF PEER REVIEW

### Basic Principles

Two strains of thought in contemporary ethical theory
have been applied to basic issues of medical ethics, yielding
two very different outcomes. The first is exemplified by
Ramsey (1970) in his book, *The Patient as Person*, in which
he defined the "covenant" between physician and patient as
the basis for ethical principles of practice. This covenant
requires both parties to maintain the sanctity of life, and
establishes caring and respect for the person as the basic
moral obligation of the physician in making individual
medical decisions and establishing rules of medical practice. The covenant is the basis of the traditional fiduciary
system of the physician—patient relationship, in which the
patient puts trust in the physician's ability and willingness
to make crucial decisions and perform vital procedures on
the patient's behalf. In this system, the physician's obligation is to serve the best interests of the patient at all costs.
The key to this system is the trust the patient has in the
physician and, by extension, in the medical profession as a
whole. In this system, medical care has traditionally been
viewed as a privilege the patient earns by engaging in the

fiduciary relationship with the physician and by fulfilling the economic obligations of this relationship.

A very different conceptualization of medical ethics is contained in *A Theory of Justice* (Rawls 1971), which advances the goal of social justice as the highest good. The concept of social justice proposes to judge behavior as moral depending on whether it maximizes individual liberty, enhances fairness, and provides equal access to necessary services and commodities among all people. In this system, the physician performs an essential service to which all have a right, thus requiring the physician to strike a balance between the needs of the individual patient and the needs of the entire society. This model society, through its legal and economic systems, has a major if not dominant influence in determining the rules of medical practice and the structure of the physician—patient relationship. This is a contractual system in which the contract established by law or by an economic third party regulates the physician—patient relationship and the process of treatment. Through agreement to this contract, the physician acknowledges obligations to society and to its economic agents, as well as to the patient. The patient may still have trust in the physician and in the profession but, in addition, has a contract that defines what to expect from both. Because health care is seen as a basic right regardless of economic means, economic third parties are created by society to guarantee this right and to act as the agent in society's contract with the physician and the professions.

The fiduciary system has been the ethical, social, and financial basis of American medicine for most of our history; most physicians continue to feel strongly that medical care is a privilege, not a basic right. Beginning after World War II, and climaxing with the development of Medicare and Medicaid in the 1960s, American society moved toward the social justice theory of medical ethics. Throughout the 1970s, organized medicine struggled to adapt to this new climate and in the 1980s began to accommodate its institutions and policies to this new public consciousness.

## Consumerism

Another recent ethical development that significantly influenced the medical practice is the consumer movement.

This ethic of accountability requires that whoever dispenses goods or services to the public must assure the consumer that the needed product will be delivered in good faith. Furthermore, the consumer has recourse for complaints and questions. This is a significant departure from the traditional notion of caveat emptor, which offered the consumer only the option to take one's business elsewhere. In the health field, this accountability ethic has had subtle but pervasive influences on the physician—patient relationship. Many patients see it as a basic right not only to receive medical care but to participate in the decisions about the type and amount of care. The traditional authoritarian relationship is no longer acceptable to many patients, who insist on being fully informed about their illness and treatment options, thus participating in the decision-making process. In psychiatry, these new rights have created many ethical dilemmas about issues such as informed consent, right to refuse treatment, and confidentiality. Related to these issues are the newly developing concepts of the right to privacy and the right to forms of deviant behavior that do not harm others. In all these areas, the psychiatrist finds the patient clothed in new rights and new legal protections that impinge on the traditional style of professional practice, and that impose new ethical and legal obligations on the practitioner.

In this climate that encourages the patient to question or challenge physicians' decisions and actions, the economic third parties representing the patient have taken on the same right to question the judgment of the physician regarding the need, cost, and efficacy of treatment. Certainly, many physicians continue to question whether the consumer accountability movement really imposes an ethical responsibility rather than simply a political or economic one. The social justice theorists, whose thinking is dominant at present, would insist that society is in the process of re-defining the basic contractual relationship between the learned professions and the public. In this view, the professions have a moral obligation to provide the services desired and needed by the public, as perceived by that public, rather than simply the services that the professions are prepared or willing to give. Failure of the professions to follow the ethic of accountability may lead to extraprofessional regulation and loss of autonomy.

## Professions and the Public Trust

Since colonial times, the learned professions (most notably medicine and law) have had the privilege of regulating themselves with relatively little interference or external supervision. Medicine has maintained this traditional independence more than most other professions. The basis of this special status is the trust individuals and society have in the ethical responsibility of physicians, a trust born of the fiduciary type of physician—patient relationship. The medical profession has traditionally relied on four factors to guarantee the competence of its members: (1) the quality of medical education, (2) the requirements of licensure, (3) the threat of malpractice suits, and (4) the oversight actions of professional societies. Although the first two, education and licensure, provide a baseline for admission to the profession, even the public long ago recognized that they provide no continuing protection from incompetence or malfeasance. In recent years, malpractice suits have multiplied and have regrettably become the most potent factor regulating the quality of care, for better or worse. In the public mind, the court has become the best or even the only recourse for the injured, angry, or disappointed patient.

The professional societies have had a very mixed record in the regulation of the medical profession, and many private citizens and government officials have perceived the societies as uninterested, impotent, or simply devious. This perceived failure of the professional societies to regulate themselves has been viewed by many as due to the most base economic motives. Widespread skepticism has been expressed by critics of medicine whether it is possible for members of the profession to forego their own guild and economic interests sufficiently to protect the public. The status of medicine as the most economically privileged profession in the nation, combined with its past opposition to many popular social welfare programs, has further undermined its public image.

These issues have served to erode the public trust, the basis of the medical profession's independence. Although many citizens may regard their own physician as ethical and competent, the profession as a whole is viewed as self-serving and untrustworthy. Gibson (1977) has written of the need for medicine to show itself capable of self-discipline, able to maintain standards of professional responsibility, and thereby deserving of the public trust. He states: "In my judgment, it is our professional responsibility to strengthen our own systems of quality assurance, show that external regulation is only minimally necessary, and thereby reaffirm the public trust." This is not simply a public relations problem or a matter of political expediency; it must become an ethical commitment of each physician.

## GENERAL CONSIDERATIONS

Peer review places certain ethical demands on both the physician doing the review and on the physician whose case is under review. When the process is part of an insurance claims review program, such as the one operated by the American Psychiatric Association, the insurance company or other third party requesting the review also has certain ethical responsibilities. This section will outline some of these ethical responsibilities involving each of the three parties involved in the peer review of insurance claims.

The physician who agrees to participate in peer review must recognize that his or her allegiance lies with the principles established by the professional association's contract with the fiscal third party. In this contract, the association agrees to provide an objective, informed, professional opinion concerning the appropriateness and medical necessity of the treatment being reviewed. Thus the reviewer's obligation is really to the profession itself and its credibility, rather than to the patient, the treating physician, or the fiscal third party. The reviewer must avoid the temptation of identifying with and protecting the physician. Likewise, the reviewer must be mindful of the natural feeling that the patient deserves every opportunity for treatment and support, even if the treatment is neither necessary nor effective nor covered under the patient's contract with the third party. The reviewer must also be aware of a tendency to protect the patient against the large, impersonal, and rich third party. The reviewer is not being called on to make a moral judgment about whether the patient deserves treatment, but rather is being asked to make a technical, professional judgment about the need for and effectiveness of the treatment according to the terms of the contract. The reviewer must also be aware of personal biases in favor of certain forms of treatment (e.g., long-term psychotherapy or hospitalization) that may make it difficult to give an honest opinion on such a case. Any physician who cannot be objective about these issues or who does not see the review process as an important professional responsibility should not volunteer for the role.

As in any type of peer review, the physician reviewer has an obligation not to review cases in which there has been personal involvement and which involve physicians who are close friends or associates. Of course, the reviewer must maintain the confidentiality of any records seen, and must recognize that this confidentiality also extends to the physician as well as the patient.

The physician undergoing review has a responsibility to submit accurate treatment reports. The falsification of records or case reports to protect the patient's access to treatment undermines the credibility of the profession itself as well as the individual physician. One of the basic ethical obligations of all physicians must be the willingness to submit one's work to review by one's peers. A deliberate effort to subvert this process is a serious ethical violation. It is also unethical for the physician to collude with the patient to obtain, fraudulently, insurance reimbursement to which the patient is not entitled.

The fiscal third party has a responsibility to maintain the confidentiality of everyone involved in the review process, the physicians as well as the patient. The third party must be willing to accept the decisions of peer reviewers and to honor its contracts with the patient and the professional association organizing the system. Thus the third party must be willing to give its policyholders those entitled services when peer review determines them to be appropriate and necessary.

## PEER REVIEW AND ETHICS ACTIONS

In the hospital setting, it is possible that serious violations of professional ethics discovered during peer review may be referred to an in-house ethics committee or one within a professional association. However, the American Psychiatric Association's (APA) peer review of insurance claims maintains anonymity of both patient and physician, so such reporting would be impossible. Even the APA does not know either name, thus preventing a reviewer from initiating an ethics action on the basis of a peer review report. Third-party payers are unlikely to initiate an ethics action since they are not directly involved in the unethical activity. It is clearly the purpose of the APA and the fiscal third parties to utilize peer review solely for the purpose of evaluating quality of care (medical necessity and appropriateness) and not as a means of regulating or monitoring psychiatric practice in any other way. There is neither the intention nor the mechanism to use claims peer review to initiate ethical actions against the physician in the case.

## LEGAL DIMENSIONS OF PEER REVIEW

As the medical profession has recognized the need for effective self-regulation and the development of providers within hospitals and professional societies to accomplish this, a body of legislation and case law has evolved to encourage and protect this process. There is general agreement that physicians are best suited to judge the competence of other physicians and the quality of medical care. Public policy has always favored protecting the activities of medical professions, which are intended to improve the standards of practice, the level of physician competence, and the quality of care. Statutes in every state have legislated this protection in varying degrees. In almost every case involving a conflict between peer review and the possible injury to individuals resulting from review, the courts have provided peer review systems with as much immunity and protection as possible as long as the process can be shown to promote higher standards of medical care. In case after case, courts have affirmed that public policy favors as much freedom as possible for members of professional peer review committees to act in the public interest and provide maximum protection for the records of such committees.

Despite these broad assurances of protection, physicians who engage in peer review have a number of recurring questions about their legal liability, such as:

• Will I be liable for a breach of a patient's confidentiality?

- Will peer review records be accessible to parties in malpractice actions?
- Can I be required to testify in court regarding a case I review?
- Can I be sued by another physician for defamation or interference in professional practice?
- Can I or my professional association be sued for an antitrust violation?
- Can I or my professional association be sued by a patient whose coverage is terminated?

In this section, we shall address these and other concerns about legal problems in peer review, particularly from the perspective and experience of the APA's peer review program. Other types of review that may have a more critical impact on a physician's professional standing (e.g., review conducted by a hospital or a credentials committee) will be discussed in less detail.

## BREACH OF CONFIDENTIALITY

The confidentiality of psychiatrist–patient communications is one of the cornerstones of the therapeutic process and a separate chapter in this book deals with the steps taken to preserve confidentiality in the peer review process. However, a number of questions remain about the liability that may be incurred by a psychiatrist who discloses confidential information to a peer review committee.

We must begin with a recognition that the traditional inviolability of patients' confidential communications has been eroded by a number of legal and economic factors. Medical records have become important sources of evidence in a wide variety of personal injury, malpractice, and divorce and child custody cases. The growing availability of life, accident, and health insurance has also introduced a major change in the status of medical records; insurance carriers and other third-party payers routinely require patients to authorize disclosure of sufficient medical information to process claims. In cases of psychiatric hospitalization, it is now commonplace for third parties to obtain the entire hospital record. The case law in this area clearly establishes the right of third parties to require such information as a condition of processing claims, as long as the information is not used for any purpose other than claims review. Since a professional society's peer review program, such as that of the APA, is acting as the agent of the third-party payer when conducting reviews of insurance claims, the psychiatrist who releases information to the third party for purposes of peer review is no more liable for violation of confidentiality than when releasing information strictly for internal review by the third party. When review is conducted using a coding system that does not disclose the patient's name, case law has provided further protection from liability for the treating psychiatrist. Furthermore, case law has emphasized that since review is performed by physicians who are aware of the confidential nature of the information, and there is little likelihood of its indiscriminate use, the physician releasing the information to a peer review committee is highly unlikely to incur any liability.

## LIABILITY FOR DEFAMATION

Physicians involved in peer review may be concerned that statements about a case under review may be considered defamatory to the physician who delivered the treatment, and thus cause a civil suit. Defamation is defined as the injury to a person's reputation by causing unpleasant feelings or opinions about the person or significantly diminishing the person's public esteem, respect, or good will. A defendant in a defamation suit has a complete defense if the statements were made in good faith and without malice, and if there is reasonable or probable grounds for believing the statements to be true. A further defense against a charge of defamation exists if the subject matter of the statement is one in which the author has a personal or public duty of a legal, judicial, political, moral, or social nature, and the statement is made to a third person who has a corresponding interest or duty.

Thus common law appears to provide adequate protection against defamation charges if the peer review process is carried out in good faith, without malice, and with proper concern for the truth. In fact, all 50 states and the District of Columbia have enacted legislation offering varying degrees of protection from civil liability to persons involved in medical peer review as long as the criteria of good faith and lack of malice are met. Some states provide absolute immunity from all civil actions related to peer review; the remainder offer a qualified immunity specifically from defamation suits. As a general rule, these statutes protect from liability not only the physician members of hospital or medical society review committees, but also protect individuals who provide information to such committees, consultants, or employees of such committees.

Courts have interpreted the three criteria of good faith, absence of malice, and reasonable effort to ascertain truth in such a broad way that these statutes provide a very high degree of immunity to a physician who engages in organized peer review. It is clear that an error in judgment or an honest misinterpretation of facts by a physician performing peer review will not undermine immunity. It is also clear that if a physician whose case is being reviewed should suffer some injury to his or her reputation, the physician does not have cause for civil suit unless malice, bad faith, and reckless disregard for the truth on the part of the reviewer can be proved. This statutory immunity has effectively removed suit for defamation as a concern for physicians or medical societies doing peer review.

## INTERFERENCE WITH PROFESSIONAL PRACTICE

Related to the issue of defamation is the question of whether a physician whose case is being reviewed can bring suit for interference in his or her professional practice and livelihood. The right of a physician to practice the profession is fundamental, and case law has protected this right from malicious interference by others. Since the key to any such law suit is proof of malicious intent, the statutory immunity for peer reviewers appears to provide the same level of protection as it does for defamation cases. It is difficult to imagine a case involving a charge of interference due to a reviewer's malice or bad faith, given the experiences of the APA's peer review system.

## DISCOVERY OF PEER REVIEW RECORDS

A major source of concern for physicians on both sides of the peer review process is whether the records of hospital or medical society review committees can be subpoenaed for use in a malpractice case. This is much more likely to be a concern for hospital review committees than for the type of review done through the APA because hospital peer review more likely focuses on cases that have developed problems or complications rather than on routine reviews often triggered by the length of treatment.

In the absence of statutes or state court decisions that specifically exclude them, peer review records can be subpoenaed for purposes of pretrial discovery. However, 33 states have statutes that provide protection against such discovery. In the remaining 17 states, discovery of these records does not necessarily mean that they will be admissible as evidence since courts must rule on admissibility of evidence on a case-by-case basis. Many higher state courts have set precedents that exclude peer review records from admission as evidence because of public policy grounds even in the absence of exclusionary statues. Furthermore, many courts have held that peer review committee reports are hearsay evidence and therefore not admissible.

In a major decision in this area, the Federal District Court for the District of Columbia stated about the peer review process:

> To subject these discussions and deliberations to the discovery process, without a showing of exceptional necessity, would result in terminating such deliberations. Constructive professional criticism cannot occur in an atmosphere of apprehension that one doctor's suggestion will be used as a denunciation of a colleague's conduct in a malpractice suit (Bredice v. Doctor's Hospital, Inc. 1970).

## LIABILITY FOR ANTITRUST ACTION

Members of hospital and medical society peer review committees have had concerns about possible law suits on the basis of antitrust charges. To maintain an antitrust action, a physician would have to show that the activities of the review committee affected interstate commerce as defined by the Sherman Act. The physician must show that the committee actually conspired to restrain medical practice or hospital operations so as to monopolize interstate commerce. This has traditionally proven a serious obstacle to a successful antitrust action and to date no case has been reported in which a physician successfully sued another physician on antitrust grounds arising out of participation on a peer review committee.

The insurance industry has, under federal law, had a limited exemption from antitrust actions to enable insurance companies to cooperate in ways essential to the business of insurance. The professional peer review of insurance claims was also initially thought to be exempt from antitrust action for the same reason. However, a recent Supreme Court decision held that professional peer review did not share the antitrust exemption of the insurance industry (*Union Labor Life Insurance Co. v. Pireno* 1982). Although this opens the possibility that a medical society review committee, or the society itself, could be sued for an antitrust violation, the problems in proving conspiracy to restrain or monopolize professional practice make it highly unlikely that such a suit would be successful. The fact that the APA's peer review system is merely advisory to insurance companies, is conducted anonymously, and does not review fees would make it very difficult to label it anticompetitive. Therefore, concern about antitrust actions against the system or its participants appears unwarranted.

## LIABILITY TO SUIT BY A PATIENT

A concern expressed by some peer reviewers and by physicians whose cases are being reviewed is that a patient whose insurance benefits are terminated as a result of peer review may sue either physician. The extensive experience with hospital utilization review has failed to produce any cases of action against a physician performing the review. Since the patient has a contract with the insurance company, any action resulting from loss of benefits would be against the company, and not the hospital or physician. There is no record of successful actions against an attending physician by a patient whose hospitalization benefits have been denied or terminated as a result of utilization review. Since the APA's peer review system is concurrent and retrospective but does not lead to a retroactive denial of benefits, patients do not experience economic loss that could be the basis for legal action against either the attending or the reviewing physician. Thus it seems clear that this type of peer review offers little likelihood of a law suit against a reviewing physician by a patient.

## SUMMARY

The legislatures and courts have increasingly recognized the significant contribution that medical peer review makes to the public welfare by improving the quality of care and avoiding unnecessary utilization. This has resulted in a growing body of legislation and case law providing protection for those who engage in peer review and eliminating the threat of civil liability.

## REFERENCES

Bredice v. Doctor's Hospital, Inc., 50 F.R.D. 256. (D.C. Dist. Col., 1970)

Cecil R: Cecil-Loeb Textbook of Medicine, 13th ed. Edited by Beeson PB, McDermott W. Philadelphia, Saunders, 1971

Gibson RW: Professional Responsibilities and Peer Review in Psychiatry. Report of a conference conducted by the APA on 11–12 March 1977. Washington, DC, 1977

Ramsey P: The Patient as Person. New Haven, Yale University Press, 1970

Rawls J: A Theory of Justice. Cambridge, Mass, Belknap Press, 1971

Union Labor Life Insurance Co. v. Pireno, 102 S.Ct. 3002, June 28, 1982

# 4

# The Politics of Peer Review

*James Egan, M.D.*

# The Politics of Peer Review

Peer review is fundamentally a political enterprise as much as it is a psychiatric one. In this regard, I refer to politics not in terms of the more pejorative aspects of the word, but in the same vein as Visher (1971), who suggested that it refers to "attempts to define the good society, to influence and define the moral and public weal, to establish concepts of conduct and responsibility for social interaction, and to chart accurately the realities of power and purpose." Similarly, Garber (1971), in his presidential address to the American Psychiatric Association (APA), suggested that "neither as citizens nor as an organized profession can we avoid 'politics' in such contexts." It is rather in the tradition of mediating among opposing forces, and the forging of a consensus for action, that I suggest peer review is largely a political undertaking.

It is clear that as a profession we are increasingly accountable, and it would seem that Schulberg (1976) is correct when he notes that "instead of assuming the initiative, mental health professionals generally respond in a reactive way to pressures for greater quality control. More stringent standards are usually adopted only after dubious practices evoke adverse publicity." Thus the major impetus for peer review came from legislation passed in 1972 in the Social Security Act, which mandated Professional Standards Review Organizations (PSROs). In response, the APA appointed two task forces on peer review, which became the forerunners of the current Committee on Peer Review. Thus, even in its origins, peer review was politically conceived.

In 1972, the APA approved a Position Statement on Peer Review in Psychiatry (American Psychiatric Association 1973). The statement noted that

> The crisis is particularly acute in relation to cost, quality, availability, and delivery of psychiatric services. . . . Each district branch therefore is expected to have a peer review organization. Such an organization should be made up of at least three knowledgeable members who represent varied experiences and approaches to the practice of psychiatry.

Implicit in the foregoing is the recognition of powerful competing forces within the profession and the expectation that by structuring the committee as suggested, conflicts can be reduced.

Although the courts have tended to move toward a national standard of practice in determining malpractice, the peer review process has tended to emphasize the local or regional nature of psychiatric practice. This apparent inconsistency can best be appreciated when one views it as a political decision. It is an attempt to reduce the tension among psychiatrists of different interests and theoretical schools. It is an effort to reach a compromise between those who are primarily invested in hospital versus office practice, or psychoanalysis versus behavioral treatments, or electroconvulsive therapy versus neuroleptics, or group versus individual psychotherapy, and so forth. By having a large, diverse, and local group of reviewers, it is believed that the possibility of getting a "bad" review at the hands of someone who is unfamiliar with one's orientation, or worse, hostile toward it, is reduced.

Another intraprofessional political obstacle to peer review concerns confidentiality. How is a patient's treatment to be reviewed by a group of local psychiatrists while maintaining complete and total protection of the patient's privacy? What information can safely be given to third-party intermediaries or to the APA's Office of Peer Review? Shwed et al. (1979) summarized this concern:

> *Third-party insurers, whether private or government, armed with computers and data banks, have seemingly insatiable appetites for detailed information about what transpires between doctor and patient in order, they say, to justify the benefits they pay, and to be assured that competent medical service has been rendered. What are the boundaries between the right to know, and the doctor's time-honored pledge to patients of confidentiality."*

Liptzin (1974) approached the problem somewhat differently when he stated that "no one is convinced that the data collected by a PSRO can be kept confidential."

Perhaps because of such concerns, considerable efforts were expended to devise a system of review that would assure privacy. The Mental Health Treatment Report, used in the peer review system of the Civilian Health and Medical Program of the Uniformed Service (CHAMPUS) and adapted by commercial insurers, was carefully designed to provide a minimum of identifying data while providing adequate information for a review. In addition, a number of efforts at all levels of the review process have been implemented to assure confidentiality. One of these is the Psychiatric Coding System of the APA. To date, no breach of confidentiality in the review process has been reported to the APA Committee on Peer Review.

A different set of concerns confronts the peer review program in its dealings with the fiscal intermediaries. Here the political struggle was between the profession and the third party intermediaries. In general, there was apprehension that the Peer Review Committee would rubber stamp the actions of the professional. From the psychiatrists' point of view, insurers only wanted to use a peer review system to control costs. The mutual suspicions were gradually reduced, and a "working alliance" has been forged under the skillful leadership of Dr. Henry Altman, chairman of the Peer Review Committee (1976–1982) and his successor Dr. John Hamilton. They were joined in this delicate undertaking by Dr. William Guillette, former medical director of the Aetna Insurance Company. As one measure of the degree to which this has been accomplished, there are currently almost 30 fiscal intermediaries, including CHAMPUS, that use the APA peer review program. It is as if both the profession and the insurance carriers agreed with Chodoff (1977) that:

> *As far as the psychiatric profession is concerned, it needs to be stated unequivocally that cost control is not the only purpose of peer review. The principal reason that organized psychiatry must continue to expand its efforts in peer review is to control the quality of the practice of psychiatry in the interests of better care for individuals suffering from psychiatric disorder.*

In 1972, the APA's position statement alluded to another political factor, namely the relationship among mental health professionals: "Broadening peer review to include assessment of the complete spectrum of physician-generated psychiatric care must initially be limited in scope . . . " (American Psychiatric Association 1973). That clearly spelled out the need to evaluate all mental health services, including those of other disciplines. The American Psychological Association has its own peer review mechanism; the National Association of Social Workers (NASW) and the American Nurses' Association (ANA) have evolving review processes. Thus, when a number of carriers have asked the APA Office of Peer Review to review social workers, it agreed to do so only if requested to do so by the NASW. Careful attention to the rights and privileges of the other mental health disciplines has gone a long way toward reducing interprofessional rivalries and antagonisms. It is not surprising, therefore, that at peer review committee meetings held during 1983 and 1984, invited guests represented the peer review committees of the American Psychological Association, NASW, and ANA.

Perhaps nowhere have the political dimensions of peer review been more apparent than in dealing with a decision in 1974 by CHAMPUS to reduce benefits significantly. That decision was rescinded:

> *because from the outset APA made it clear, however, that we recognized the need at both the local and national levels to find appropriate solutions to the very real problems*

*of quality assurance and cost containment . . . . It is our
firm belief that if APA had not given its pledge to work with
CHAMPUS . . . or if this pledge had lacked credibility, the
cutbacks would have proceeded as originally planned
(Spiegel 1974).*

In less than 10 years, psychiatric peer review has
evolved from a legislative mandate to a position statement
by APA—to a fully functioning operation. Peer review has
demonstrated that it can readily meet its established objective: the professional monitoring of the utilization and quality of psychiatric care. The implementation of the APA's peer
review system represents the successful outcome of many
political compromises.

## REFERENCES

American Psychiatric Association: Position statement on peer review in psychiatry. Am J Psychiatry 130: 381–384, 1973

Chodoff P, Santora P: Psychiatric peer review: the Washington,
D.C. experience, 1972–1975. Am J Psychiatry 134:2,
121–125, 1977

Garber R: The presidential address: the proper business of psychiatry. Am J Psychiatry 128:1, 33–43, 1971

Liptzin B: quality assurance and psychiatric practice: a review.
Am J Psychiatry 131:12, 1374–1377, 1974

Schulberg H: Quality-of-care standards and professional norms.
Am J Psychiatry 133:9, 1047–1051, 1976

Shwed H, Kuvin S, Baliga R: Medicaid Audit: crisis in confidentiality and the patient-psychiatrist relationship. Am J Psychiatry 136:4A, 447–450, 1979

Spiegel J, Hammersley D: Peer review: an obligation for psychiatrists (editorial). Am J Psychiatry 131:12, 1382–1384,
1974

Visher J: Some Criteria for Political Involvement. Unpublished
paper read at the Trustees Meeting, American Psychiatric
Association, Washington, D.C., 18 March 1971.

# 5

# Psychodynamic Aspects of Peer Review

*William Offenkrantz, M.D.*

# Psychodynamic Aspects of Peer Review

This section is written primarily for medical doctors outside the field of psychiatry and persons interested in health care problems entirely outside the field of medicine (e.g., health planners, legislators, insurance company executives). Consequently, some of the material will be familiar to the psychiatric reader. For this larger audience, some historical descriptions and definitions already familiar to psychiatrists may be in order.

Peer review has been a traditional part of medical education, especially in small group teaching in the years of the medical students' clinical clerkships. The same experience continues during psychiatric residency training and throughout our medical careers, whenever we choose (or are required) to present our patients or the descriptions of our treatment to colleagues in whose hands we are willing to trust our self-esteem, thus returning us to student status. It is during this sequence that the obvious positive psychodynamic effects of peer review are most noticeable. It increases our sense of professionalism in both cognitive and emotional ways, especially as it offers us perspectives on our work from points of view beyond or at least outside our own. In addition, it promotes healthy identification with respected colleagues. It is also at these times that we learn to tolerate the temporary return to a student or con-

81

sultee status for the sake of striving for greater professional competence, often referred to in intrapsychic terms as our professional ego ideal. This requires us to consider any "graduation" exercise as the doorway to new learning, rather than as a rite of passage to a land where our hard-won credentials are all we need to avoid further scrutiny.

The conscious anxieties connected with this process are usually described as stemming from an examination of our work (usually experienced as fear of being judged inadequate) or loss of income if our work is judged as inappropriate. Similarly, our patients must tolerate conscious anxiety about loss of privacy (never total, but hardly ever experienced as trivial) connected with knowing that their doctors, as part of their training or continuing education, are presenting the treatment to colleagues. However, as will become clear from the definitions that follow in this section, I will not be dealing with the conscious anxiety about adapting to the practical reality of third-party payments requiring both patient and psychiatrist to sacrifice some of their privacy, both as individuals and in their relationship with each other. Instead, this section on psychodynamics will be about the partially or totally unconscious meanings that such a situation may have for the parties involved. It should be emphasized that the fact of these meanings being psychodynamically (rather than simply descriptively) unconscious does not necessarily imply the presence of a neurotic process.

It has been suggested that one source of concern associated with peer review comes from the psychiatrists' awareness that something new, different, and special is being done (R. Michels, personal communications, 4 April 1983). All of the anxieties that may occur in such a situation are as likely to strike patients as well as doctors when the peer review procedure is also sudden and unexpected. Thus the classic determinants for overwhelming psychological trauma may be present.

In the mid 1970s, 75 percent of American psychiatrists who participated in field trials for the official diagnostic nomenclature of the American Psychiatric Association (APA)—the DSM-III (American Psychiatric Association 1980)—defined themselves as psychodynamically oriented (Cooper and Michels 1981). What is it that is customarily meant by such a self-designation, and how is it applicable to the psychodynamics of peer review?

Psychodynamics, as generally used in psychiatry, refers to a set of inferences about mental life that are close enough to the data of clinical observation to be readily verifiable. This even applies to those psychiatrists who are devoted to phenomenology and other descriptive approaches in their effort to avoid premature conclusions about the etiology of mental disorders.

The psychodynamic point of view is sometimes thought to include obligatory reference to psychic "energy" and psychic "structure," both characteristic of psychoanalytic metapsychology. However, in this section, it refers specifically to the following set of assumptions: (1) the existence of unconscious mental activity, (2) the important ways in which behavior is often determined by factors outside our conscious awareness, and (3) the important manifestation of this determinism by the effect of early life experience on adult attitudes, behaviors, and perceptions (Offenkrantz and Tobin 1974). More precisely, the vicissitudes of maturation and development have a lasting effect on behavior; the adaptations made during each developmental stage affect the stage that follows (Lewis and Usdin 1982).

For those readers not accustomed to psychiatric clinical interviews as a source of data about mental life, the following examples may be useful. The first and second assumptions may both be demonstrated by the phenomenon of posthypnotic suggestion, in which a normal person may behave in a strange way, determined by a factor outside the person's awareness. Similarly, the first two assumptions are also illustrated by a patient with a passive–aggressive personality disorder who is unwittingly subject to "forgetfulness," in a "resistance to demands for adequate performance in both occupational and social functioning" (Spitzer 1980, p. 186). At a more complicated level, patients who have compulsive personality disorders typically display isolation of affect. This means that they are unable, in the psychiatric interview situation (as in the rest of their lives), to experience simultaneously powerful affects and the ideas connected with them. This observation, although intimately related to the psychodynamic concepts of unconscious wishes, unconscious fears, and unconscious defense mechanisms, can nevertheless be made reliably on the basis of clinical observation. These defense mechanisms involve an unconsciously active mental process, called repression, by which such a person responds to the conflict between a wish and the fear it stimulates in a way that results in important aspects of thinking, feeling, and decision making becoming psychodynamically unconscious (i.e., not available to awareness by volitional introspection) (Lewis and Usdin 1982). The third assumption, about the effects of early environmental experience on adult life, seems well-enough understood and accepted, both in and outside of psychiatry, so that no further examples are necessary.

There are other definitions that will facilitate the understanding of peer review's psychodynamics. We begin with the definition of intrapsychic conflict. This concept follows from the basic premise that the mind is not unitary and that its parts may enter into conflict with each other. In everyday language, one may be "of two minds" about something. In motivational terms, this refers to the simultaneous presence of incompatible goals, one or both of which may be experienced unconsciously *or* consciously. These goals often involve a fantasied or real gratification, whose attainment entails what the person unconsciously believes is a significant threat to one's security. A conflict is considered a symptom when it is repressed (as defined above), and when one or more of the conflicting goals is inappropriate to the age and circumstances of the person, such as the goal being symbolically elaborated from an earlier age. Thus neurotic symptoms may be an expression of one's effort to resolve such painful conflict when one or both of the conflicting ideas are unconscious. The symptom then may simultaneously reflect the wish to gratify an impulse, to punish oneself for the forbidden gratification, while remaining unaware of either side of this transaction.

A typical example of such a neurotic symptom is an hysterical neurosis of the conversion type in which a loss of physical functioning results from unconscious intrapsychic conflict in which both the wish and the fear are being symbolically elaborated from an earlier age (American Psychiatric Association Committee on Peer Review 1981).

The experience of needs and wishes (desires) begins very early in life and is intimately related to the childhood experience adults call the "frightening expectation of danger," when those needs and desires are inevitably not satisfied in time to keep inner tension from rising in the mind or body of the child. These frightening expectations arise in a manner parallel to the motivational systems. This means that all behavior is designed to fulfill needs originating at various levels of development. These needs range from basic biologically determined ones (e.g., attachment to the parenting person) to those that express complex goals and values (e.g., willingness to die for a cause). Thus behavior can be understood as motivated, generally tending to avoid (psychic) pain, and maintaining pleasure, interpersonal security, and self-esteem (Lewis and Usdin 1982).

What are some of these typical danger situations? It follows from the preceding paragraphs that, in order to understand the intrapsychic conflicts that may occur in the peer review situation, we need to identify the typical early-life anxieties, the derivatives of which may still be present. These can be described in the following oversimplified, albeit accurate, way. They generally occur as part of a series of developmental tasks and are capable of being dealt with in average expectable ways, leading to symptom-free adult life by the time the developmental crises associated with puberty are mastered. First is separation-individuation, in which the child's anxieties are related to the tasks of emerging from a symbiotic fusion with the mother (separation) and of assuming one's own individual characteristics (individuation) (Mahler et al. 1975). These tasks should be completed by about 36 months of age, in conjunction with the child's ability to maintain a relationship in one's own mind, even with someone who is absent for a relatively long time.

Second is the development of a cohesive sense of self: composed of the blending of our tamed infantile grandiosity into mature ambition, along with the tamed infantile exaltation of our parents into mature enthusiasm for our leaders. The anxieties associated with these developmental tasks occur between birth and about six years (Kohut 1977).

During the same period of time as the two foregoing sets of tasks and their associated anxieties are occurring, we find the following additional anxieties regarding:

1. Loss or separation from a person on whom the child depends for love and care (associated with the task of

developing basic trust in another person's love and reliability);
2. Anger or disapproval from such a person;
3. Physical punishment for transgressions real or imag-
ined;
4. Punitive conscience (guilty disapproval of ourselves
when we transgress parental prohibitions);
5. Shame, feelings of humiliation, or feelings of inferiority
based on disapproval by significant others or ourselves,
for not living up to our ideals.

The second and third anxieties are associated with the task
of developing a sense of self-control and autonomy.

A final important definition is that of transference,
which refers to inappropriate perceptions, attitudes, desires, feelings, and qualities of interpersonal interaction
that an individual tends to create in relationship to significant people. These distortions reflect past experiences and
ongoing needs imposed on current relationships, which are
often markedly discrepant with the realities of the relationship. They are unconscious repetitions and displace-
ments of reactions stemming from significant relationships
of childhood.

For the sake of simplicity, I will sacrifice precision in
regard to such concepts as countertransference, and will
group together all distortions, whether by the patient, the
psychiatrist, the peer reviewer, or the third-party payer. The
major determinant of distortion in the peer review process
is the situation within the mind of the patient and/or the
psychiatrist, and/or the peer reviewer, and/or the person
perceiving the treatment on behalf of the third-party payer.
Peer review is the occasion for their elaboration and not
their cause.

I suggest that these distortions may occur in addition
to those described earlier as the average expectable fears
about peer review: sudden, unexpected novelty; concern
about being found inadequate; loss of income; and loss of
privacy. The behavior of the doctor, patient, reviewer, or
third-party payer may be defined as psychopathological
when it:

1. Causes conscious distress to the individual (i.e., "symptoms" occur); or

2. Is maladaptive and inflexible, thereby inhibiting the capacity for pleasure, self-fulfillment, and optimal functioning; or
3. Brings the individual into self-conflict or conflict with the environment (e.g., by imposing unnecessary suffering on others) (Lewis and Usdin 1982).

There are few reports in the literature on the psychodynamic effects of insurance reimbursement processes on psychotherapy and psychoanalysis (Halpert 1972a, 1972b). The most complete description of these issues (including the patient's and psychiatrist's psychodynamic reactions to the peer review process and to the third-party payer) is contained in a case report by Rudominer (1981). It describes the case of a patient successfully treated by psychoanalysis over a 4-year period. It is especially interesting from the standpoint of illustrating a mental mechanism from the separation-individuation phase, called splitting. In this patient's mind, the third-party payer was experienced as "a mother figure, a dispenser of nourishment," and the peer review process, as a "depriving parent." She experienced great difficulty before she could integrate the two images and experience the "good" and "bad" parents as part of a single entity. Other reports about the psychodynamic aspects of peer review typically deal with the patient's and the psychiatrist's anxiety and resentment about loss of privacy and, in the psychiatrist's mind, the fear of appearing incompetent (Chodoff 1972; Gottesman 1972, 1974; Kass et al. 1980; Luft and Newman 1977; Luft et al. 1976; Newman and Luft 1974).

## PSYCHODYNAMIC ASPECTS OF PEER REVIEW FROM THE PATIENT'S VIEWPOINT

The range of patients' experiences with peer review covers the entire spectrum of psychodynamic possibilities that have been defined above. For illustrative purposes, I will select the most common reactions by following the various developmental tasks and their associated anxieties as they are reexperienced in the treatment situation.

The patient may experience peer review as a threat to a basic sense of trust in the transference figure that has come to be relied on: the psychiatrist. If the patient is reexperiencing in therapy the developmental tasks of separation and individuation with the psychiatrist, the presence of a peer reviewer or third-party payer may be experienced as a threat to the symbiotic tie that precedes the patient's ability to (re)discover individual characteristics.

If the patient is reexperiencing in therapy the developmental task of achieving a cohesive sense of self, in order to restore a loss in self-esteem, the patient may temporarily be using the psychiatrist as a "mirror," affirming a still-alive, childhood grandiosity; or as someone to idealize, as a child who sees the parent as all-knowing and all-powerful. In such situations, the presence of the third party may disrupt the existing mirroring or idealizing transference because the patient feels the psychiatrist's empathy for his or her needs, on which a vulnerable self-esteem depends, is destroyed by this third party.

In a way that derives from a later developmental state, the patient may experience guilty fear about the revelation of how he or she has transgressed parental prohibitions by expressing hitherto unacceptable feelings in the presence of an approving authority figure: the psychiatrist. Although self-esteem has risen during the therapy, the patient may feel threatened by peer review or the third-party payer, just as was felt toward the psychiatrist at the beginning of treatment: a threatening, punitive, authority figure.

Another relevant developmental experience during peer review is the patient's history with multiple, simultaneous authority figures and the loyalty problems that may have arisen at such times. This is especially true if, as a child, the patient learned to deal with anxieties by setting one parent against the other. The patient can relive that experience by setting the psychiatrist against the peer reviewer or the third-party payer. For example, the patient may attempt to enlist the psychiatrist in collusion against the third party or peer reviewer as "the other parent" against whom the patient and psychiatrist unite. Similarly, the patient may experience the psychiatrist as a sibling and invite the psychiatrist to unite against both "authoritarian parents": the third-party payer and the peer reviewer.

It is not surprising that one of the more common reactions of patients to peer review is related to their anxiety about exhibiting themselves and being looked at. This is a common enough experience for many children who have played some version of "the doctor game" and learned about sexual anatomy with a mixture of excitement and apprehension. This same mixture of feeling stimulated and being afraid of exposure is frequently present in the minds of patients whose treatment is being "looked at."

All of the foregoing psychodynamic findings conform to the usual ways in which psychiatrists think about how the presence of *any* third party becomes grist for the treatment mill. There is one other finding, however, that is less familiar to the profession. It is the situation that occurs when the patient cannot comprehend the actual constructive quality of the psychiatrist's relationship with whomever the third party may be. This is difficult for a patient to comprehend, in the same way the patient often had difficulty understanding the true nature of his or her parents' interaction with each other. This difficulty, when the patient was a·child, was partly due to a lack of cognitive maturity, but more importantly, was due to the patient's primitive emotionality. The patient turned the parents' ordinary, everyday interactions with each other into age-appropriate fantasies such as those involving violence or primitive sexuality. This was accomplished according to the unconscious formula: "If I can't understand what they are doing, I'll make them be like me." Then the child no longer feels left out of the parents' interactions because the child identifies with either the aggressor or the victim (Offenkrantz and Tobin 1978). This is similar to the way in which patients in treatment with student psychiatrists regard their doctor's relationship with a supervisor as a primitive one, and then identify with either the student or the teacher, in order not to feel left out. Likewise, patients have difficulty believing their psychiatrist is not submitting obsequiously, dominating with arrogance, or appearing willing to cheat in the relationship with the third party.

## PSYCHODYNAMIC ASPECTS OF PEER REVIEW FROM THE PSYCHIATRIST'S VIEWPOINT

Any or all of the developmental tasks and anxieties that were described for patients may occur with psychiatrists as well, especially those related to being looked at and exhibiting oneself.

In addition, the doctor is more likely to have anxiety about the peer reviewer, which may stir up earlier-life competitive struggles: either with siblings or with the parent of the same sex. Thus the psychiatrist may join the patient in a sadistic fantasy that "we will cheat the insurance company together," or the opposite, masochistic fantasy that "we are the helpless victims of this powerful external force" (Pulver 1976).

Psychiatrists are also accustomed to the autonomy that comes with solo medical practice. This autonomy, contributing to pleasure and pride in their work, may be perceived to be at risk and cause anxieties about loss of control. When asked, psychiatrists most often cite "exam taking" as the cause of their anxiety about peer review. Furthermore, they also make reference to their early-life experiences with fear of physical punishment from their parent of the same sex, for hostile feelings that the future psychiatrist felt in the familiar triangle known as the family romance.

If a patient with disordered self-esteem experiences the psychiatrist in the transference as an affirming (mirroring) echo of grandiosity, or as an idealized, all-powerful parent, then the psychiatrist's ability to remain empathically in touch with the needs of such an extremely taxing patient may be compromised by the psychiatrist's preoccupation with his or her *own* self-esteem. The psychiatrist may only recognize the signal of this reaction when becoming bored or otherwise unresponsive to the patient's demands.

For psychiatrists, as well as for all other human beings, the developmental stage of desexualized interest and concern between two adults who meet regularly alone together over a long period of time and listen to one of the two reveal their most intimate secrets, is a difficult level to achieve and to maintain. When we fill out an insurance or peer review form at the beginning of treatment, it is an act not just for the patient and not just for ourselves. Ideally, it represents for both psychiatrist and patient an expression of the unique intimacy and the tender concern characteristic of the psychiatric treatment situation we know is about to unfold. It is because of our conflicts about making this **explicit to ourselves that psychiatrists may perceive the presence of *any* third party in a regressed, primitive way.**

## PSYCHODYNAMIC ASPECTS OF PEER REVIEW FROM THE THIRD-PARTY PAYER'S VIEWPOINT

Members of society in general, third-party payers, and many members of the medical profession view psychiatrists as practicing in mysterious ways (GAP Committee on Therapy 1978). This attitude reflects an "outsider's" fascination with, and fear of, the "dark side" (i.e., the unconscious aspects) of their own minds. Insisting that psychiatrists practice mysteriously is a way of avoiding confronting and understanding the everyday existence of unconscious attitudes in themselves. To the extent that psychiatrists enjoy this exalted status as "keepers of the secrets," they are encouraging the expression of the depreciation that inevitably follows such exaltation. For their arrogance, these psychiatrists must be willing to pay the price commonly expressed in derogatory jokes about them.

One psychodynamic problem faced by third-party payers' medical directors is their identification with the practicing psychiatrist and loyalty to the profession versus loyalty to one's employer. On a more abstract level, this problem can become acutely painful when the tension is between the goal of cost containment and the goal of quality control.

## PSYCHODYNAMIC ASPECTS OF PEER REVIEW FROM THE PEER REVIEWER'S VIEWPOINT

Once again there is nothing entirely new here that was not also described as a potential problem for patients as well. What is new is that the peer reviewer is in the position of a potentially powerful judge, even though the reviewer's opinions are usually advisory and there is almost always a group of two to three reviewers. Still, intense competitive conflicts from early-life experiences with siblings or parents can be stirred up by being a peer reviewer . Direct expressions of aggression may surface, or unconscious defenses against such impulses may predominate (e.g., reaction formations such as rescue fantasies directed toward the practitioner). These may take the form that the practitioner "needs to be educated," or may be directed toward the patient who "needs to be saved from an (incompetent) practitioner." The

quotation marks are used to indicate that these are distorted perceptions, based on the peer reviewer's own earlier-
life conflicts. In addition, loyalty conflicts between allegiance to a fellow practitioner and to the agency paying the
peer reviewer may be stimulated in a way that rekindles old
sibling rivalries and parental loyalties.

The peer reviewer may have a psychodynamic conflict
that is the other side of the coin of the psychiatrist's wish
and fear about exhibiting one's work and relationship with
the patient. That is, the reviewer may be in conflict about
looking at this uniquely intimate relationship between two
other adults.

Finally, a brief note about a treatment plan for these
varied psychodynamic conflicts, at least insofar as the psychiatrist and the patient are concerned. This "treatment"
depends on the type of therapy the patient is receiving. In
the realm of the psychodynamically oriented therapies, the
APA's book on *Treatment Planning in Psychiatry* (Lewis
and Usdin 1982) lists five forms of psychotherapy. In the
supportive forms it is common to use psychotherapy in
conjunction with medication. It is also not rare to use medication in symptom-relief-oriented psychotherapy as well.
However, apart from the indications for medication, the
psychiatrist must decide whether and (when appropriate)
how much of the psychiatrist's understanding of the patient's reaction to peer review should be made known (interpreted) to the patient.

In the case of those patients who have difficulty with
reality testing, it is important to decide also how much of
the psychiatrist's *own* psychodynamic conflicts about peer
review needs to be shared with the patient. Here, as in all
other instances of the interpretation of psychological conflict, the first step is to inform the patient of the presence of
anxiety in his or her behavior. Next, the psychiatrist interprets what the patient does when anxious by naming the
defense in everyday language. Third, the nature of the anxiety is interpreted. Finally, the psychiatrist interprets the
possible sources of gratification in the same behavior that
was also motivated by anxiety. For example, a woman patient may experience peer review with anxiety at being
"looked at." She may wish that the analyst, experienced as
mother, will defend her against the intrusive scrutiny of the
peer reviewer, experienced as her father. Only later should

the stimulation and possible gratification of being looked at by father be brought from the past into the here-and-now situation involving peer review.

In conclusion, I would offer a suggestion to psychiatrists as a group (Offenkrantz and Tobin 1978). As psychiatrists, we constantly struggle to achieve the psychiatric ideal of the most highly integrated ways of dealing with various tensions, thereby enabling us to treat our patients properly in pursuit of healing and truth rather than some form of infantile gratification for ourselves. However, the inevitable facts are that as individuals we do not always achieve this ideal, nor does our psychiatric group always live up to its own ideals. When this happens, we become vulnerable to more primitive forms of relief of our various anxieties, both with our patients and in relation to other psychiatrists.

It is my conviction that we can achieve this goal of treating our patients properly and pursue truth only by the mixture of mutual support and confrontation engendered by frank discussions of the psychodynamics of peer review with other psychiatrists in small groups.

## REFERENCES

American Psychiatric Association: Diagnostic and Statistical Manual of Mental Disorders, 3rd ed. Washington, DC, American Psychiatric Association, 1980

American Psychiatric Association Committee on Peer Review: Manual of Psychiatric Peer Review, 2nd ed. Washington, DC, American Psychiatric Association 1981

Chodoff P: The effect of third party payment on the practice of psychotherapy. Am J Psychiatry 129:5, 540–545, 1972

Cooper A, Michels R: Review of Diagnostic and Statistical Manual of Mental Disorders, 3rd ed. Am J Psychiatry 138:128–129, 1981

GAP Committee on Therapy: Psychotherapy and Its Financial Feasibility within the National Health Care System (Research Rep. No. 100). New York, Group for the Advancement of Psychiatry Publications, 34, 1978

Gottesman D: Peer review: what are we afraid of? New Physician: 21:611, 1972

Gottesman D: Measuring attitudes about peer review in a university department of psychiatry. Hosp Community Psychiatry 25:39–41, 1974

Halpert E: A meaning of insurance in psychotherapy. Int J Psychoanal Psychother 1:62–68, 1972a

Halpert E: The effect of insurance on psychoanalytic treatment. J Am Psychoanal Assoc 20:122–133, 1972b

Kass F, Charles E, Buckley P: Two years follow up of a peer review training program for residents. Am J Psychiatry 137:244–245, 1980

Kohut H: The Analysis of the Self. New York, International Universities Press, 1977

Lewis JM Jr, Usdin G (eds): Treatment Planning in Psychiatry. Washington, DC, American Psychiatric Association, 1982

Luft L, Newman D: Acceptance of peer review in a community mental health center. Hosp Community Psychiatry 28:889–894, 1977

Luft L, Sampson L, Newman D: Effects of peer review on outpatient psychotherapy: therapist and patient follow-up survey. Am J Psychiatry 133:891–895, 1976

Mahler M, Pine F, Bergman A: The Psychological Birth of the Human Infant. New York, Basic Books, 1975

Newman DE, Luft L: The peer review process: education vs. control. Am J Psychiatry 131:1363–1366, 1974

Offenkrantz W, Tobin A: Psychoanalytic psychotherapy. Arch Gen Psychiatry 30:5, 593–606, 1974

Offenkrantz W, Tobin A: Problems of the therapeutic alliance: analysis with simultaneous therapeutic and research goals. The International Review of Psychoanalysis 5:224, 229, 1978

Pulver S: Survey of psychoanalytic practice. J Am Psychoanal Assoc 26:626–630, 1976

Rudominer H: Peer review, third-party payment, and the analytic situation: a case report. J Am Psychoanal Assoc 32:4, 773–795, 1981

Spitzer R: Quick Reference to Diagnostic Criteria from DSM-III. Washington, DC, American Psychiatric Association, 1980

# 6

# Peer Review from the Perspective of the Third Party

*William Guillette, M.D.*

# Peer Review from the
# Perspective of the Third Party

E arly group health insurance policies excluded maternity and psychiatric care as areas that would be too
expensive to insure. The maternity exclusion has all
but disappeared over the years, but very few policies provide
open-ended psychiatric benefits. Most policies have a dollar
limit, a hospitalization limit, and/or a substantial co-pay-
ment requirement for office therapy. Health insurance policies reimburse for the treatment of diseases and accidental
injuries, providing the treatment is customary, reasonable,
and medically necessary. A service or supply is considered
necessary only if it is broadly accepted professionally as
essential to the treatment of the disease or injury. In psychiatry, as opposed to other branches of medicine, there are
few objective indicators (e.g., radiology, laboratory tests)
that validate medical opinions about diagnoses, response to
treatment, and severity of illness (Fowler 1978). In the past,
the psychiatric profession has been criticized for imprecise
diagnoses and the lack of good criteria as to treatment and
determination of recovery.

The American Psychiatric Association's (APA) criteria
sets are a major step forward to assist in reviewing level of
care needs for psychiatric patients. Claims personnel are
not qualified to make judgments as to the necessity and
appropriateness of care; this can only be done by psychia-

trists. Thus, to arrive at fair and reasonable judgments as to what is necessary care and to discourage unorthodox practice, the third-party payer must have the cooperation of well-qualified and respected physicians who are willing to participate in quality peer review programs for both outpatient (office) and inpatient care.

The purpose of peer review is to assure quality care, with neither overutilization nor underutilization of medical services. Cost effectiveness is a by-product of good peer review. Peer review is a potent tool that will affect the standards of practice in a community, but it requires the cooperation of all providers. It requires the commitment of time by professionals whose time is valuable. In return for this commitment, they must be assured that their efforts will not be wasted and, thus, they must have enough "clout" to ensure the success of the program. Peer review should be part of a total quality assurance program that is applied to current cases as well as retroactive reviews. This includes educating providers, when necessary, as to standards of care, both through the monitoring of processes and outcomes.

Peer review usually means a review of the written word; that is, the provider's report or the hospital's record. According to Fowler (1978), the lack of appropriate documentation of the need for care is probably the most frequent reason for denial of payment by a third party. This is so, both for outpatient and inpatient care.

## OUTPATIENT CARE

Reports on outpatient care are usually very skimpy and frequently neglect to state:

- the specific diagnosis,
- the cause of the symptoms,
- the need for psychiatric treatment,
- the goals of treatment,
- the expected length of treatment,
- the justification for the frequency of visits, and
- the prognosis.

This type of information should be provided to the carrier on the special report form developed by the APA. In most cases, it will obviate the need for requests for additional information and will result in timely processing of the claim.

## INPATIENT CARE

Reviewing claims for inpatient care differs from reviewing office therapy. The patient's problem must be such that hospitalization is medically necessary. If the patient can be treated as an outpatient or at a lesser level of care, then hospitalization is not indicated.

The APA's "Model Screening Criteria Format for Inpatient Treatment" should be used as a guide (American Psychiatric Association 1981).

In most cases, the psychiatrist has overall control of the case. All the services provided to the patient must be prescribed and directed by a physician. The physician is the kingpin of therapy, guiding the members of the therapeutic team—including the psychologists, social workers, occupational therapists, group therapists, nurses, attendants—who work directly with the patient. The physician writes the orders for therapy and is responsible for evaluating the therapeutic program. The physician determines what progress, if any, has been made and whether treatment goals are realistic or whether different therapy is indicated. The physician must have direct contact with the patient on more than a "Good morning, nice to see you" basis and must meet with the other professionals on a regular basis to discuss the case. The prescribed treatment must be reasonable for that particular patient, and the record must document what is going on.

In cases involving short-term confinements, a report form may contain sufficient information for review purposes. In cases of prolonged hospitalization, more information is usually needed and the hospital record becomes very important. In most cases, this is the document that determines coverage, unless the physician elects to send a narrative report that contains the needed information. Thus the staff must write legibly and document delivery of appropriate treatment for each condition requiring care.

Six crucial questions that should be addressed on the hospital record are:

- Why is the patient in an acute hospital setting at this time?
- What are providers trying to do for this patient?
- How do they plan to do it? Is the treatment appropriate?
- How is the patient doing? Has the patient attained the maximum benefit from hospitalization?
- Could this patient be treated at a lesser level of care?
- Is this custodial care?

Other factors are:

- Timeliness of procedures,
- Frequency of progress notes (at least twice a week),
- Use of staff conferences, and
- Use of overnight, daytime, and weekend passes.

The written record is a reflection of what has happened and, as we all know, some people write better than others. Regardless, providers must realize that they will be judged by the quality of the record. In the medicolegal area, there is an old adage: "Work not written is work not done" (i.e., if it isn't in the record, it will be considered in court as never having been done in the first place, even though the witness says, "I always do a rectal exam").

## WHAT SHOULD THE RECORD INCLUDE?

1. *History*
   What symptoms or behavior necessitated the current admission?
   What was the mental status on admission?
   What factors contributed to the present illness (environmental, internal, or dynamic)?
   Has the patient been in treatment before?
   What was the previous treatment (treatment setting and type/frequency of interventions)?
2. *Treatment Goals*
   Do the goals foster the patients' return to his or her highest level of adaptive functioning or reconstruction?
3. *Therapeutic Plan*
   What was the frequency and duration of all therapies and by whom?

Are the therapies used considered "generally accepted" by the profession?

What medication is being given?

Who is directly responsible for the care and management of the patient?

What was the frequency of the supervision?

4. *Patient's Response to Therapy*

Is there documentation supporting the patient's response to therapy (e.g., such comments as "continued depression, suicidal, responding to treatment, not responding to treatment")?

5. *Consultation Reports*

Are consultation reports attached or referenced in the treatment report or medical record?

6. *Special Studies*

Were special diagnostic tests conducted?

If so, are results documented?

7. *Discharge Summary*

Is there a comprehensive discharge summary, containing statements as to what led to the hospitalization, treatment, progress, and patient's condition on discharge?

Also, comments on abnormal lab findings or normal findings on special tests and a statement as to postdischarge plans (i.e., where is the patient going and what is the patient going to do) are appropriate.

Prompt reimbursement is not usually a problem when there is adequate documentation as to the reasonableness and necessity of the case.

The APA's peer review program is an excellent example of how the insurance industry and the psychiatric profession can work together to assure that mental health insurance remains a viable health benefit.

## REFERENCES

American Psychiatric Association: Manual of Psychiatric Peer Review, 2nd ed. Washington, DC, American Psychiatric Association, 1981, pp. 22–29

Fowler DR: The psychiatrist and health insurance claims review. J Clin Psychiatry 39:519–522, 1978

# 7

# The CHAMPUS Psychiatric and Psychological Review Project

*Alex R. Rodriguez, M.D.*

# The CHAMPUS Psychiatric and Psychological Review Project

Among the key developments in the evolution of psychiatric peer review in the United States was the implementation of a national system of retrospective review of psychiatric services provided under benefits coverage by the Civilian Health and Medical Program of the Uniformed Services (CHAMPUS) of the Department of Defense. As a major health benefits program, CHAMPUS occupies a unique place among third-party payers in that it has multiple constituencies and must fulfill many roles and functions. Multiple forces brought the American Psychiatric Association (APA) and American Psychological Association into collaboration with CHAMPUS to create the first major national peer review activity. These same forces continue to shape this important demonstration of the capacity of a professional organization and third-party payer to provide cooperatively for quality and cost-beneficial psychiatric care. This chapter will trace the development of this project, review the outcomes to date, and provide thoughts about the future directions that appear likely to evolve in project activities.

## OVERVIEW OF THE CHAMPUS PROGRAM

CHAMPUS was originally implemented by an act of Congress in 1956, in part to provide for supplementary medical care for dependents of active personnel because of evident limitations in health care services provided at military treatment facilities in the wake of the Korean War. Support for complementary civilian medical services grew in the ensuing years from many groups. The military services found that CHAMPUS coverage of their beneficiaries allowed them to orient greater proportions of their professional health care resources to active service members' health needs and associated military readiness missions. Military families were satisfied with the greater health care options that civilian services provided and with the quality of care. Retired military eyed these expanded services longingly and used the growing strength of their organizations to promote expansion of CHAMPUS coverage for them and their beneficiaries. Burgeoning demand for health care services at military treatment facilities by retirees reinforced the services' support for further CHAMPUS assistance. The services also found themselves in lagging competition for skilled personnel who were required to utilize the increasingly more sophisticated military technologies and who were being lured into the civilian work force by attractive salaries and benefits. With ensuing growth in the national economy, the federal government, health insurance and health benefits programs, and public sector entitlement programs, the momentum soon gathered for expansion of the CHAMPUS benefits program. Thus, these forces consolidated in 1966, shortly after creation of the Medicare program, to drive the creation of P.L. 89-614 (Military Medical Benefits Act of 1966), which established the basis for the current CHAMPUS program and the CHAMPUS regulation (Department of Defense 1977).

Modeled by law after the Blue Cross High Option Plan, the progression of benefit and reimbursement policies over the ensuing years has tended to follow the directions set by national Blue Cross and Blue Shield policies. In addition, CHAMPUS has tended to parallel policy developments by the Medicare and Federal Employee Health Benefits Program, since they share common identities as federal health benefits programs. CHAMPUS has tended to be reactive in incorporating policies developed by these various programs, due to its limited staff developmental resources and its concept under enabling legislation. Nevertheless, it has found itself having to break new ground from time to time according to the expressed interests of its multiple constituency groups—primarily Congress, the military services and Department of Defense, active duty and retired services members' organizations, and national health care provider organizations.

The net result of their interests and efforts in the past has been progressive and selective expansion of program benefits to the point that current benefits are among the most broadly covered of any comparable employee health care plan. This growth has resulted in program costs escalating from $435 million in 1973 and $591 million in 1978, to the fiscal year 1984 budget of approximately $1.4 billion—during a time of phenomenal expansion in the health care industry (Office of Civilian Health and Medical Program of the Uniformed Services 1984). This growth has been characterized by increased health services' availability and escalating health care costs associated with such elements as inflation, sophisticated management services, and technological developments. As all third-party payers have been affected by these increased health care costs in a profitable and proliferating provider and technological market, efforts have consistently been directed toward implementing quality control and cost accountable systems—primarily as a basis for reimbursement. Thus such terms as *quality assurance* and *utilization review* were born to encompass a multitude of health services' review activities that have become an elemental part of the superstructure of current and future health care in the United States. The growth of these activities in the late 1960s and 1970s—particularly as promulgated by the larger third-party payers such as Medicare—set the direction for programs like CHAMPUS, especially as they proved effective and became part of the routine business practices imposed by third-party payers on health care providers. It was in this evolving scenario that CHAMPUS found itself cast into an unanticipated but unavoidable course of action that would undeniably alter its program and national health care itself.

## THE RESIDENTIAL TREATMENT CENTER CRISIS AND THE SELECT COMMITTEE ON PSYCHIATRIC CARE AND EVALUATION

Among the benefits adopted by CHAMPUS during its growth in the late 1960s was psychiatric care of children and adolescents in residential treatment centers. This benefit was created originally in recognition of the high demand for such care by military communities, which generally provided limited or no intensive or comprehensive psychiatric services for children and adolescents. In creating the benefit, however, CHAMPUS was unable to regulate residential treatment centers other than requiring state licensure for CHAMPUS certification. In turn, individual states had few guidelines other than basic facility structural and safety requirements. Thus, lacking any national admission, treatment criteria, or program standards for such a diverse number of psychotherapeutically oriented residential centers, CHAMPUS soon found itself paying some $20 million per year by 1974 to approximately 486 recognized facilities, which ranged in quality from the academically affiliated and professionally staffed centers to those that, at best, were board and care facilities.

Like other third-party payers, CHAMPUS' means of assessing the medical necessity of rendered care was limited to its few professional criteria and reviewers. Under such circumstances, it is not surprising that there were real problems due to the lack of federal and state controls that had traditionally monitored the quality of care of these psychiatric facilities. However, what was unexpected was the seriousness and magnitude of the problems that resulted.

In the summer of 1974, the nation was shocked to discover that there were serious outright abuses of patients' rights in several residential treatment centers, and often basic therapeutic services were not rendered (Wooden 1976). In short order, the Permanent Subcommittee on Investigations of the U.S. Senate Government Operations Committee, under the direction of Senators Henry Jackson and Charles Percy, opened hearings in which CHAMPUS was called to account for its lack of awareness and control over these situations (U.S. Senate 1974). CHAMPUS was directed to take definitive steps to remedy the problems. At this moment of truth, the Department of Defense took a direction that was to change the way that the program and many third-party payers were to conduct business in the future.

The easy path for CHAMPUS might have been to terminate the benefit, with the justification that quality controls over residential treatment center services were not possible. This could have been justified by the view of other third-party payers that reimbursement for residential treatment center care was risky because of its high costs and problems in routinely assessing medical (psychological) necessity through claims and infrequent professional reviews. However, the Department of Defense considered the needs of military families and the impact of terminating the benefit on military communities and military health care facilities (Penner 1975).

In a departure from its usual autonomous and reactive approaches to policy development, CHAMPUS turned to the professional community for assistance in developing a quality assurance plan for its residential treatment center benefit. In September 1974, CHAMPUS entered into a cooperative agreement with the National Institute of Mental Health (NIMH) to establish the Select Committee on Psychiatric Care and Evaluation (SCOPCE). This activity received the support and assistance of the APA, which had been one of the medical specialty societies that had provided early leadership in focusing professional organizations' attention on the developing fields of quality assurance and utilization review (American Psychiatric Association 1975). The project was described as:

> a pioneering effort for the mental health field: the first multidisciplinary mental health peer review ever undertaken on a national scale, and the first system to employ such innovations as unannounced site visits to enforce its own rigorous sets of standards, prescreening and pre-authorization for payment, and contractual participation agreements with each facility (Asher 1981).

This initial SCOPCE project developed the facility and therapeutic program standards and admission and treatment criteria that were not only to affect residential treatment centers that wished to do business with CHAMPUS, but also were to provide a model for professional quality assurance.

In the vigorous and successful efforts that have followed this initial focus on residential treatment centers, CHAMPUS has been able to provide continuing refinement of the standards-criteria and effective review of services provided and billed (Margolis J, McDermott J, Vaughn W: Peer Review for Residential Treatment Centers: A Collaborative Effort of the American Psychiatric Association and CHAMPUS. Unpublished manuscript, 1983). The net result has been a sharpened definition of the residential treatment center level of care, establishment of reasonable cost controls through professional determinations of such factors as appropriateness of admission and length of stay, and the maintenance of a needed service for military families. Significanctly, CHAMPUS and its professional collaborators were able to establish quality control mechanisms over a level of service that most third-party payers and many government administrators thought was uncontrollable and undefinable.

The productive outcomes of this enterprise were of interest to many because of the unique marriage between the insurance business and professional claims that traditionally had been so often alienated from and distrustful of one another. The experience that CHAMPUS gained led it to engage the NIMH further in efforts that resulted in the development of concurrent review criteria and procedures for inpatient psychiatric care of schizophrenic adults and retrospective peer review of psychiatric inpatient services. An analysis of these latter efforts indicated that demonstrable improvements occurred in the quality of care through the professional monitoring of services and that professional review yielded a benefit-cost ratio to CHAMPUS of at least 25:1 (Sorensen J, Zelman W: CHAMPUS Experiences with Concurrent Peer Review: Case Studies, Utilization, and Cost-Effectiveness Analysis. NIMH unpublished manuscript, 1980).

Such significant financial consequences were unanticipated and caught the attention of many who were initially skeptical that the professions could make recommendations that might result in reductions in program costs. The prevailing bias was that quality assurance and quality of care activities were exercises that would inevitably expand services and concomitant costs, since it was in the financial interests of the professions to do so. These initial results were an interesting twist and a confirmation that professional ethical standards about medically (psychologically) necessary care superceded purely economic incentives. It became clear to the mental health professions that it was in their ultimate interests, economic and otherwise, to establish standards for normative and acceptable professional practices (so the outcomes were not particularly surprising to them). However, the cost data were obviously of great interest to providers since it reinforced their contention that they were the best qualified persons to make determinations about medical (psychological) necessity. If the upshot of all of these revelations and realizations was not immediate, it soon became clear that this would either become a marriage made in heaven or in hell. As CHAMPUS embarked on incorporation of the professions into its operating modes, the professions began the tender transformation toward assisting third-party payers do their business—including restricting and denying services.

## THE EVALUATION OF PEER REVIEW AT CHAMPUS

During the years of the SCOPCE projects (1974–1979), a number of situations were developing nationally that would influence CHAMPUS, other third-party payers, and administrative and professional entities. The primary promoters of these changes were national recessionary and inflationary trends, the increased availability of medical services, increased public and private sector-generated health care coverage, and increased numbers and types of health care providers. These phenomena resulted in a multitude of services and rapidly escalating costs of care that threatened to inundate third-party payers' capacity to assess and pay for medically (psychologically) necessary services.

With the prospects of depleted financial resources with which to pay for services, third-party payers were faced with either arbitrarily cutting benefits, increasing cost-shares and premiums, or increasing management initiatives that would protect benefits by providing for both effective

therapeutic and resource controls. Quality assurance activities were seen as an essential approach for the management of health care services. Utilization review activities
grew out of concomitant management requirements for
quality control of health care utilization and cost by normative and cost-benefit-defined practice standards. These
parallel activities frequently merged in program design and
implementation so that often quality assurance and utilization review were functionally inseparable.

Since quality assurance activities primarily were the
province of health care professionals and utilization review
activities were the province of health services and systems'
managers, the overlapping roles sometimes created inter-
authority conflicts and role ambiguity. In such situations, it
became difficult for practicing professionals to trust the
infusion of cost-consciousness and cost-containment into
quality of care definitions and standards, and similarly difficult for resource managers to trust the cost growth poten-
tion of those same quality of care definitions and standards. The uneasy alliances that developed made for uneven
performance that has characterized many of the fusion
quality assurance-utilization review activities, such as hospital utilization review committees required by the Joint
Commission on Accreditation of Hospitals, professional
standards review organizations established for the Medicare program, and health systems agencies established for
local health resources management.

Despite these problems, it became inescapable for both
the professions and resource managers that they not only
had to coexist but that they had to coexist in a trusting
relationship and with common goals. It was just such a
growing trust that led CHAMPUS—through relationships
developed in the SCOPCE experiences—to develop cooperatively a novel peer review project with the APA and American Psychological Association.

## DEVELOPING THE CHAMPUS PSYCHIATRIC AND PSYCHOLOGICAL PEER REVIEW PROJECTS

Among the developments of the SCOPCE projects that demonstrated to CHAMPUS the quality of care and cost benefits
of professional input for their health benefits determina-

tions were professional and peer review activities. Psychiatrists, psychologists, and social workers were recruited through NIMH and by professional associations and contracted to provide team reviews of admission and continuing care indications for children and adolescents admitted to residential treatment centers. Psychiatrists identified by NIMH and the APA assisted with concurrent review of psychiatric admissions for treatment of CHAMPUS beneficiaries admitted with the diagnosis of schizophrenia to civilian hospitals in the San Diego, California, and Norfolk, Virginia, areas. These activities provided an indication to CHAMPUS that there were resource management and patient care accountability benefits in systematic peer review. Although third-party payers such as CHAMPUS had retained professionals to conduct case reviews for many years, such arrangements had tended to be irregular, oriented toward exceptional case circumstances, only occasionally structured to allow review by a person of similar professional training as the health care provider, and viewed by providers as review conducted by "hired guns" rather than true peers who would represent true professional interests.

Over time, a concept of peer review developed within SCOPCE in which CHAMPUS would contract directly with national mental health professional associations to provide case review. The potential advantages of such an arrangement for CHAMPUS were:

1. The development of professional review resources that could advise the agency on the medical (psychological) necessity of care being provided by an ever-expanding mental health community and for conditions and treatments that were not easily understood or accepted by the third-party payer community;
2. The maintenance accountability about mental health benefits and costs, by collaborating with recognized national authorities to develop state-of-the-art treatment criteria; and
3. The containment of costs associated with unnecessarily prescribed or lengthy care.

The initiation of a peer review system was a good-risk arrangement for CHAMPUS because its success could solve many of its dilemmas while failure would provide further guidance on how better to manage mental health benefits. Furthermore, the blow would be softened for CHAMPUS because it would be a joint failure guided by the incompetence of the mental health field. On the other hand, the risks and hurdles were decidedly higher for the professional associations and the advantages were seemingly fewer. No doubt many psychiatrists and psychologists thought their leadership had taken leave of their senses and betrayed professional interests by colluding with parties who advocated the questioning of their professional judgment, possibly resulting in the restriction of patients' access to them.

While accurately sizing up the formidable tasks of selling this peer review arrangement to its membership and developing a system that would function effectively, the leadership of the APA and American Psychological Association was astutely gauging the future challenges that lay in the mental health professions' path if they didn't begin to develop some evidence that mental health services were definable, accountable, and efficacious. Collaboration with CHAMPUS provided the APAs an opportunity to develop a program with a unique beneficiary-oriented mission, experience working with other national mental health organizations, and national visibility. Furthermore, the program size was not so large as to present operational problems in setting up a pilot project, or so small as to minimize the potential gains for so significant a commitment. Moreover, it is also apparent that the professional associations were guided by professional practice standards, decisions regarding appropriate patient care, and the general moral conduct of the profession. These were all seen as issues that were girded by an arrangement in which the professional associations were actively involved.

Thus, in July 1977, the Department of Defense signed contracts with the APA and American Psychological Association to develop a national system of psychiatric and psychological peer review. Although it was almost 2 years before the APA, the American Psychological Association, and CHAMPUS would actually begin peer review activities, that time was needed to lay the standards and procedural groundwork for peer review operations and to gain the professional support that would be absolutely necessary for the project to succeed. Among the significant concerns raised during the development period were the following:

1. Whether the professional criteria and standards that were to be adopted for review would adequately allow for acceptable variances in professional therapeutic approaches and not reflect theoretical biases;
2. The types of built-in protection to ensure confidentiality of the patient-client, therapist, and reviewer;
3. The provisions made for reimbursement of the therapist for time spent in completing a mental health treatment report;
4. The ensuing legal ramifications for the therapist and reviewer as a result of unfavorable review conclusions; and
5. The guarantees provided by CHAMPUS that recommendations would not violate antitrust laws.

These were pithy issues requiring early resolution through much thoughtful formulation, consensus-building, and careful monitoring (Rodriguez 1983).

During the period of 1977–1979, a number of tasks needed to be completed in preparation of peer review. Each association had to establish administrative offices, national advisory committees, review protocols, and review criteria for use by CHAMPUS claims processors and peer reviewers. Although the APA developed a *Manual of Psychiatric Peer Review* (American Psychiatric Association 1976) in recognition of third-party payers' need for professionally developed treatment guidelines, a manual specific to the CHAMPUS psychiatric benefit was needed, incorporating updated psychiatric standards, reporting formats, and procedures relevant to CHAMPUS peer reviewers and psychiatric services providers (Office of Civilian Health and Medical Program of the Uniformed Services 1980a). The American Psychological Association developed its own manual after it was decided that differences in professional therapeutic and diagnostic approaches would make the formulation of a joint manual a difficult task.

Some 350 psychiatrists were identified as peer reviewers from each district branch and were trained in CHAMPUS' peer review procedures. Special provisions were made with the American Academy of Child Psychiatry and American Psychoanalytic Association to identify peer reviewers with specialized certification in child-adolescent psychiatry and psychoanalysis and to develop special review criteria for treatments provided by such specialists. During this development phase and prior to the initiation of peer review, a number of provider-oriented briefings and publications were promulgated by the APA to promote understanding of the system, solicit recommendations, and provide assurances that potential problems were being attended to by the APA, the American Psychological Association, and CHAMPUS.

All parties understood that peer review activities would add time to claims processing and, in some instances, might result in partial approval or full denial of care. Balanced against potential cash flow problems and possible lags in therapeutic processes were the benefits of having peers conduct a more objective and thorough review than might be provided by insurance company nurse reviewers. Furthermore, adverse decisions were subject to a second APA peer review by means of CHAMPUS' reconsideration and appeals system.

Many providers remained very uneasy about providing privileged information to a third-party payer, despite these professional protections. In addition, many felt that there were basic problems inherent in any document-based review system that linked to variables of information validity, completeness, and formulation; to treatment criteria representing norms of practice; and to the subjective judgments of reviewers. Although none of these issues could be completely controlled, there were some checks provided, such as the provision of three reviewers per case to minimize reviewer variability. Although there may have been some level of cooperation based on resignation during the early developmental stages of this project, the prevailing attitude of the professions, peer reviewers, and many psychotherapists was that the implementation of CHAMPUS' peer review system would ultimately benefit the professional associations, practitioners, and patients.

## EARLY EXPERIENCE WITH THE PEER REVIEW SYSTEM

A number of previous articles have commented on various aspects of peer review as it relates to the CHAMPUS project

(Claiborn et al. 1982a, 1982b; Cohen 1981; Cohen and Holstein 1982a, 1982b; Cohen and Nelson 1982; Cohen and Oyster-Nelson 1981; Cohen and Pizzirusso, in press; Offenkrantz 1982; Rodriguez 1983; Snipe 1980; Stricker 1982; Stricker and Cohen 1983). Although this chapter will not detail the observations or conclusions of those publications, a summary of selected key points will be made about the project's initial experiences. In general, several lessons have been learned from both the successful and problematic areas of the system that should provide some guidance for any future planning and applications of peer review. Total yearly costs have averaged approximately $2 million to CHAMPUS for review services and administration of some 1,800 outpatient psychological, 2,500 outpatient psychiatric, and 2,100 inpatient psychiatric cases yearly—or approximately $150 for three reviews per case, including administrative costs (Rodriguez 1983). These reviews have resulted in the dispositions shown in Table 1.

These outcomes have resulted in approximately $6 million in outright documented cost avoidance to CHAMPUS over a 2-year period (1981–1982), although Rodriguez (1983) believes the actual costs savings would be much higher if the peer review "sentinel effect" could be calculated. This might not seem like a significant figure for a program that has seen psychiatric and psychological benefits costs escalating at rates approximating 25 percent per year and that spent over $170 million in 1982 for psychiatric–psychological care. It might also not seem very exact, and it is not. When the peer review project was established, a sophisticated cost-benefit evaluation component was not

**Table 1.**  Peer Review Determinations 1981-1984

|  | Approvals (%) | Partial Approvals (%) | Denials (%) |
|---|---|---|---|
| Outpatient Psychological | 47.5 | 46 | 6.5 |
| Outpatient Psychiatric | 53 | 38 | 9 |
| Inpatient Psychiatric | 60 | 27 | 13 |

designed and incorporated into data collection. In retrospect, such a component should have been included, even given the methodological problems with extracting data, drawing conclusions, and CHAMPUS' limited information systems resources.

In general, however, some observations can be made, for which there is admittedly little exact data. During the 2-year period of 1981–1982 and the initial 5 months of fiscal year 1983, it appears that the rates of cost increases for inpatient psychiatric costs (hospital and professional) were less than those of inpatient medical and surgical care. For whatever reasons this might be, at least one factor that has to be considered is that of the peer review sentinel. CHAMPUS has no such peer review monitor for nonmental health inpatient or outpatient care. However, third-level (medical) reviews are occasionally conducted when unusual claims data are kicked out of lower-level reviews (automated and by nurse and nonprofessional reviewers). Medical and surgical costs have tended to be held down somewhat in areas where CHAMPUS has also had pilot contracts with effective Professional Standards Review Organizations (PSROs). However, the exact cost savings are difficult to ascertain, given the cost models used thus far. All of this suggests two things:

1. More exact cost-benefits models need to be developed and implemented into peer review systems; and
2. Given current data, it appears peer review results in at least modest cost savings.

Of course, with employment of more exacting review standards-criteria and monitoring, greater cost avoidances would be expected. With CHAMPUS' generally broad psychiatric–psychological benefits during the initial phase (1977–1982) and a reimbursement policy that pays billed charges on a local UCR ("usual, customary, and reasonable") basis, it should not surprise anyone that program costs have escalated, with or without a sentinel. The author believes that much of the cost-avoidance that might be accrued in peer or other professional review systems is minimized by such open-ended reimbursement policies. For this reason, it is likely that many third-party payers will continue to find both prospective reimbursement and review systems attractive. The likely directions that will be taken will be discussed subsequently in this chapter.

In addition to the costs consequences of peer review, a number of other observations can be made about the early experiences.

## Improved Quality of Patient Care

Peer and other professional review activities have been shown elsewhere to improve quality of care and clinician performance (Deuschle et al. 1982; Sinclair and Frankel 1982). Since the peer review project established no means of objectively measuring changes in quality of care, it has clearly and strongly been the consensus impression of APA peer reviewers, APA administrators, and CHAMPUS professional staff that documented care has significantly improved. However, the greater measure of progress has been in the care reflected in medical judgments associated with evaluations and treatments—with greater attention shown to practice within established standards of care in the United States.

It is well accepted that quality care is cost effective over the long run, by reducing complications and other consequences of inappropriate and inadequate care (Sharfstein 1982). Thus CHAMPUS may well accrue cost savings from its beneficiary population over time as a result of improved quality of care in the current phase of treatment provided under its peer review activities. Some practitioners might question if denial or partial approval of treatment might have not only negative longitudinal therapeutic consequences but also costs consequences. Although there might indeed be individual circumstances where such negative consequences have occurred, they have not been identified to the APA or CHAMPUS or demonstrated to be solely the result of the peer review itself. Therefore, taken as a whole, CHAMPUS is satisfied thus far that psychiatric and psychological treatments are at least of a quality that would be consistent with regulatory and professional requirements of medical (psychological) necessity—even if the costs for that and all other health care continue to increase at alarming rates.

## Increased Professional Involvement with Peer Review

When the peer review project began, there was limited individual and collective professional commitment to its function and success. While the leadership of the APA and American Psychological Association clearly supported the project, several state and local professional organizations remained either neutral or negative toward it. It was a novel and unproven activity that posed potential problems for practitioners' incomes and traditional practice autonomy. However, with increasing acknowledgment of the real future of peer review as reflecting both professional and third-party payer interests, practitioners and their local professional associations are showing at least greater interest in, if not actual support of, peer review activities. Attendance at state and national association-sponsored continuing education and training sessions on peer review is notably and consistently greater than in the past. Increasingly larger numbers of psychiatrists and psychologists are inquiring about participating in the project as peer reviewers and are showing an interest in bringing peer review arrangements into their local professional associations. The expression of recalcitrant and hostile attitudes has diminished considerably.

Although there may certainly be continued reasons for frustration with the system—such as challenges to peer reviewer justifications for partial approvals or denials, slightly increased delays in reimbursement, and concerns about the objectivity, validity, and specificity of the standards and criteria—nevertheless most practitioners have come to realize that peer review now represents the manifestation of a professional ethic about quality and cost-conscious care as much as it represents yet another administrative overlay to their practices. Moreover, many are beginning to develop a more forward-thinking and creative view of peer review services and the implementation of local peer supervision as components of continuing education. In all of this, professionals are beginning to respond to peer review positively, less as an instrument by which third-party payers question their judgment and morality, and more as an exercise by which peers may provide feedback that can sharpen clinical judgments and skills.

The more professional associations engage third-party payers in designing peer review systems that are of educational value to practitioners, the more relevant such systems will be to the professions and practitioners. The APA, the American Psychological Association, and CHAMPUS have initially explored the possibilities of setting up flexible systems of peer review with direct contact between mutually consenting practitioners and reviewers. Although operational and administrative considerations currently prevent the development of such a system, such unique approaches will no doubt be considered within various peer review systems in the future.

## Acknowledgment by Third-Party Payers

One of the significant consequences of recent experiences with psychiatric and psychological peer review has been the keen interest demonstrated by other third-party payers. Both the APA and the American Psychological Association have entered into numerous contracts with various not-for-profit and commercial health insurance carriers. There is currently growing momentum in the health insurance and health benefits business in not only retrospective review, but also prospective review. It is quite likely that developing arrangements between third-party payers and professional associations will continue, particularly as such associations see the benefits of developing and marketing review services. Thus far, the professions have shown they can deliver reviews that result in definitive cost-savings from unnecessary and unjustified care. As a result, third-party payers are gradually acknowledging

1. The appropriate and primary roles of professionals in making routine judgments about medical (psychological) necessity of care;
2. The role of professionals in making determinations about quality of care through development of standards of care; and
3. The need for professional guidance in establishing benefit coverage based on evolving professional acceptance of diagnostic nosologies, treatments, and levels of care.

## SPIN-OFFS OF THE PROJECT

A number of positive potential direct and indirect outcomes were anticipated by the professions—primarily related to educational and research opportunities. In addition, CHAMPUS thought there might be beneficial cost and management outcomes associated with refinements of criteria sets and review protocols and then subsequent effect on claims processing and benefit determinations. In general, these anticipated spin-offs gained the ongoing attention of the APA, the American Psychological Association, and CHAMPUS, but the nature of the information gathered and reviewed has resulted in unanticipated attention as well. The following represent some of the areas that have required and received attention.

### Development of Educational Objectives

Both the APA and the American Psychological Association realized that they should develop and promote the educational experiences accrued from organized peer review activities. Both associations have focused attention primarily on familiarizing practitioners with the review system and training reviewers. Broader educational objectives for practitioners emanating from the review feedback have not been developed yet, but such feedback could become an important means of providing educational experiences in professionally developed evaluation and treatment standards. To date, there are unexplored opportunities in formally linking peer review experiences with continuing medical education systems. Some psychiatric district branches have pursued active independent peer review-related activities, such as publishing case review sections in monthly newsletters that contain questions and answers related to case management and cost issues, and promoting monthly "peer supervision" study groups that review cases under treatment by participants.

Such local enterprises, particularly as they respond to district branch peer review and educational goals, reaffirm the essential importance of peer review being as locally and professionally guided as possible—a principle affirmed by the House of Delegates of the American Medical Association

(AMA) in 1982 and by the APA. In addition, the APA will soon be spearheading an effort within the AMA for affirmation of the need for quality assurance peer review to be included as necessary components in medical school and graduate medical education curricula. The Association of American Medical Colleges has provided some initiative toward this early professional training with its recent publication of instructional texts in quality assurance for health professionals and trainees (Williamson 1982; Williamson et al. 1982) and a few schools of medicine and professional psychology have initiated didactic and experiential training in quality assurance-utilization review (Bent 1982). A number of professional organizations besides the APA and the American Psychological Association are increasingly recognizing the importance of providing education and training in these areas and are offering more continuing education credits at professional meetings aimed at increasing awareness and performance in quality of care and cost containment. The emergence and rapid growth of the American College of Utilization Review Physicians and the conferring of board status to the American Board of Quality Assurance and Utilization Review Physicians further demonstrates that such issues are becoming part of the recognized necessary skills in providing health care in a contemporary and future United States.

These and other pilot efforts are providing early experiences with developing the essential knowledge and skills bases for practitioners and trainees, but will ultimately require some broader directions from the professions, through formulation of profession-wide educational and practice objectives. In the future, the possession of quality assurance and utilization review skills will become essential for all health care practitioners, not only for reimbursement of services rendered but also to verify professional competence. The peer review project has demonstrated this and points to the need for both individual practitioners and their various professional associations to take some definitive and immediate steps toward developing educational objectives that are consistent with the ever-growing information requirements imposed by third-party payers and others with administrative and fiscal authorities. A "wait and see" attitude by the professions will result in such authorities becoming further alienated from and imposed on the practitioners.

## Development of Research Objectives

Like similar quality assurance—utilization review activities, the peer review project is an information-generating system. Although the value of clinical information for third-party payers such as CHAMPUS would seem to lie primarily in the function of allowing determinations to be made about medical (psychological) necessity of services, there are important opportunities to be gained linking them to actual utilization rates and concomitant costs by analyzing professional practice trends, treatment processes, and outcomes. Moreover, it would be interesting to determine if peer review alters providers' behavior, particularly in the light of development of evaluation criteria and standards, reporting formats, and reimbursement and benefit policies.

Realizing that the need for more sophisticated and structured data analysis has grown as the project has matured, the APA, the American Psychological Association, and CHAMPUS have automated the processing of peer review information and have begun strategic planning for a project evaluation component. At this writing, these activities are at an early level of development and no definitive outcomes can yet be reported.

In establishing research objectives for the project, the APA, the American Psychological Association, and CHAMPUS acknowledge that systematic and controlled data-based approaches to designing, monitoring, and analyzing project activities are essential not only to future professional objectives but also to the management of project resources. Ultimately, it is important for all to marry such data with other available program utilization and cost data, such as that previously analyzed by CHAMPUS (Office of Civilian Health and Medical Program of the Uniformed Services 1980b) and Dorken (1977). The limitations thus far in conducting such collaborative enterprises have been related to a number of situations:

1. Lack of awareness by third-party payers and professional organizations of the potential uses or importance of such data;

2. Lack of awareness by professional organizations that the data might be made available for their analysis;
3. Occasionally, lack of access to the information by researchers and professional organizations, due to proprietary or administrative concerns by third-party payers;
4. Methodological obstacles, such as assessment contamination due to incomplete or meaningless data;
5. Reluctance by the professions and third-party payers to be seen as collaborators, particularly as data steers either one to conclusions that, in the public domain, might not be in one or the other's interests; and
6. Administrative concerns, such as which party should underwrite the costs of the research.

Such research can be costly, and it seems there is some expectation in such situations that someone else should pay for it. This is unfortunate for the mental health professions, as they have missed many opportunities to gain access to data that, for a modest investment, could substantiate the essential roles of mental health services in overall health benefits and the demonstrated efficacy of psychotherapy from a cost-benefit and utilization perspective. At a time when costs of health care imperil mental health benefits, this need for data should be a concern to many. Thus both third-party payers and professional associations should be highly interested in establishing research objectives if there is any interest in demonstrating the cost benefits and efficacy of peer review and psychotherapy. The need and opportunity for collaborative research ventures is now substantial.

**Development of Professional Standards of Care**

In establishing the project, the APA, the American Psychological Association, and CHAMPUS determined that their respective professional standards of practice needed to be incorporated into documents that could guide peer reviewers and practitioners regarding acceptable practices and determinations of medical (psychological) necessity of services. The challenge was to develop standards that were specific enough to be definitive and yet broad enough not to be arbitrary or restrictive of the range of theoretical orientations and therapeutic modalities represented in the psychiatric and psychological professions. In general, the standards developed have been considered reasonable and representative of the mainstream practices in the United States. CHAMPUS' interest in this "normative" definition of professional standards is driven by its regulation, which limits reimbursement for only "medically (psychologically) necessary care," or that which is required for the evaluation and treatment of a medical (psychological) disease, illness, or condition, and which reflects the standards of care generally provided in the United States. Professional services provided for "mind expansion" or other purposes where there is not a defined mental disorder are not authorized as a benefit.

The effectiveness of the standards has been demonstrated by their consistent reaffirmation in various legal appeals, determinations, and professional appraisals, and by their adoption by other third-party payers for use in claims review. Their efficacy has steered CHAMPUS to recognize the potential roles of professional organizations in developing other such standards that are required for administration of specific benefits, such as alcohol–drug rehabilitation, psychiatric partial hospitalization, and residential treatment center services. Admission and treatment criteria, facility program standards, professional credentials, facility certification, and efficacy-safety of various therapeutic modalities have all received the attention of the APA and the American Psychological Association in their advisements to CHAMPUS.

By defining their standards, the psychiatric and psychological professions have clarified their unique and specific identities and functions. In doing so, they have both educated and relieved third-party payers, which traditionally have been particularly ignorant and distrusting of psychotherapy providers and practices. The greater refinements of such standards are already underway, and will become a major focus of interactions between the professions and health administrative–fiscal authorities in the future, in much the same manner that health care technology and therapeutic assessments are now receiving a high level of attention from various national public and private sector entities concerned with health care services and funding.

CHAMPUS, the APA, the American Psychological Association, the National Association of Social Workers, and the American Nurses' Association are already developing another first effort in this area, with their joint attempt to develop a consolidated review manual and report forms for use by psychiatrists, psychologists, social workers, psychiatric nurses, and marriage and family therapists, all recognized as authorized providers by CHAMPUS. Such efforts as this will challenge all parties in the future to ensure that care is not compromised by overrestrictive or nonspecific practice requirements. The role of third-party payers in seeking such standards from professional resources in the future will likely have a significant effect on the scope and nature of professional practices in the future—for better or for worse (Rodriguez, unpublished manuscript 1983).

### Development of Facility Survey Protocols and Standards

One of the critical actions undertaken by CHAMPUS during the SCOPCE activities focusing on problems in residential treatment centers was the implementation of a survey branch as an operational component of the Office of CHAMPUS. Using facility program standards developed by SCOPCE, the survey branch conducted hundreds of on-site surveys of residential treatment centers throughout the country. This resulted in CHAMPUS' decertification of all substandard programs and substantial improvements in the treatment programs in others.

This highly successful venture was eventually terminated when CHAMPUS decided to fulfill goals for residential treatment center authorization by requiring certification by the Joint Commission on Accreditation of Hospitals (JCAH). Thus CHAMPUS substituted JCAH requirements for routine CHAMPUS surveys. However, by the fall of 1981, it became clear from patterns of questionable practices identified through peer review of services rendered in a few psychiatric facilities that irregularities needed to be addressed. In these facilities, such practices as inappropriate admissions, excessive and unjustified lengths of stay, questionable use or nonuse of therapies, and even treatment planning and documentation were repeatedly being commented on by various peer reviewers who, by nature of confidentiality protocols, were unaware of each other's concerns or the identities of the facilities.

The National Advisory Committee of the APA recommended that on-site "quality of care" visits be reinstituted using CHAMPUS professionals and provider representatives. Subsequent site visits confirmed suspected problems and provided suggestions (consultations) that could be used by facilities to address problem areas. These visits, while understandably threatening to the facilities, were conducted with such a high degree of professional courtesy and objectivity that, in each instance, the facility considered it to their benefit. The residential treatment centers recognized it was not to their financial or professional benefit to have quality of care questions raised by CHAMPUS or any other third-party payer. CHAMPUS and the APA were concerned only that the irregularities be remedied so that beneficiaries and practitioners not be further restricted by professional reservations about rendered care. In each situation, the changes implemented have been significant and, thus far, lasting.

These experiences might have caused CHAMPUS to question the effectiveness of JCAH standards or state licensing authorities' monitoring. However, what has actually ensued is the recognition that the actual number of facilities involved has been small, problems were surmountable, and the remedies were generally within the realm of professional resolution. This should affirm several issues: (1) most facilities share a professional attitude; (2) facilities are attempting to practice within established requirements; (3) the overall quality of JCAH standards has not suffered; and (4) the peer review system was effective in identifying irregularities. Thus guidance and oversight have occurred through CHAMPUS' prospective standards and JCAH, through concurrent professional and administrative adherence to quality of care by the facilities, and by retrospective monitoring through peer review. Although the role of on-site or delegated concurrent review, such as that performed by PSROs, remains undefined as part of an overall care and cost monitoring process, nevertheless it is apparent thus far that CHAMPUS has established a relatively sensitive system of facility review. Further it is quite clear this could not have been accomplished without the professional guidance of the APA.

## Development of an Impaired Provider Program Concept

One of the dilemmas confronting third-party payers over the years has been what to do when claims information identifies practitioners whose clinical expertise and ethical standards do not conform to those prescribed by their profession(s). Generally, third-party payers' greater concerns have been related to the specific case determination of medical (psychological) necessity and whether to pay or not to pay. The predominant approach has been to encourage behavioral changes in the practitioner through nonpayment for questionable services and practices. There has been little or no tendency to accept responsibility for aberrant practices except where they were clearly illegal, or where they were consistently so extreme that the practitioner's status within a health benefits plan or community required review by an administrative or professional body. More often, professional concern has never focused on these problems, as most claims are reviewed by nonprofessionals. Medical or other professional review is generally conducted only if the reviewer is cognizant of the irregularities. Therefore, there have been limited roles and operations established by third-party payers to deal with the errant practitioner. However, this has begun to change as professionalization of third-party payers has occurred. With the use of nurse reviewers conducting second-level review, physicians conducting third-level review, and the concomitant acknowledgment that equivocal care often results in revenue loss for the payer, there is the realization that professional and administrative protocols are needed to monitor quality of care in the claims review process. Furthermore, some have realized that mechanisms are needed to intercede in instances where there are questions about the practitioner's competence.

In developing its peer review system, CHAMPUS unknowingly consigned itself eventually to confront the unavoidable evidence found in treatment reports and case files—namely, there are a few psychiatrists and psychologists who are "impaired" by virtue of a lack of evident knowledge and skills; by their inability to utilize the skills they possess; by neglecting the standards or ethics of their profession; or by their disregard of the law. This definition of impairment is broader than the state and medical associations' conventional focus in recent years. Their focus has been on certain physicians' problems with alcohol or other drug dependence or emotional problems that limit their capacity to practice medicine. The authors' concept of impairment also regards incompetent physicians and other health professionals as being compromised by other defects in addition to alcohol or other drug dependence that similarly limit their capacity to provide quality care.

Occasionally, problems identified by peer and professional reviewers can be traced to practitioners' lack of attention to records, poor organization, or patient overload resulting in an inattention to patient care details. More often, it is apparent that the practitioner simply has not developed the necessary cognitive and conscience capacities in training and continuing education to allow him or her to provide quality and conscientious care. From the third-party payers' point of view, this situation is reaching a point where there is risk to too many parties. Certainly, for the impaired provider there are legal and financial risks in subjecting oneself to peer review that could result in loss of competitive edge, financial security, or freedom. The patient is at risk financially, physically, and emotionally. The third-party payer is primarily at risk financially, but certainly could suffer legal consequences if it knowingly possessed information indicating that a patient's health was compromised as a result of poor quality care. Thus the third-party payer could also become an accomplice in instances of unfortunate sequelae due to iatrogenic causes. Finally, the attendant professional organization, as a fourth party to this compact, is also at risk because its most important responsibility is to provide society with qualified practitioners. While quality control is difficult to ensure in any business or profession, it is most expected in health care. Because of these risks, CHAMPUS and the Office of the Assistant Secretary of Defense (Health Affairs) have initiated review and planning activities that will explore the roles of local and national professional entities and administrative structures such as CHAMPUS and state licensing authorities in promoting quality assurance in health care provided under Department of Defense auspices.

These quality assurance efforts are driven not only by resource management responsibilities, but also the broader implied accountabilities involved in the covenants with military families and units to provide quality health care. In addition, the more recent infusion of professionals in health benefits management has brought professional ethical responsibilities into an arena where cost considerations have been paramount and continue to be of great concern. The merger of these developing resource and professional views will result in an increased focus on the impaired provider. It is the clear intent of the Department of Defense to engage the health professions developing mechanisms to identify, monitor, and limit the unsupervised practices of impaired practitioners. The quality assurance provided in such joint ventures can reduce risks and inappropriate expenditures that are compromising contemporary health care.

## Expansion, Development, and Consolidation

CHAMPUS is in the process of extending independent authorized provider status to clinical social workers and clinical nurse specialists. In addition, CHAMPUS has recognized marriage and family therapists as mental health providers. As a result, CHAMPUS has initiated the development of peer review systems for clinical social work services with the National Association of Social Workers, for psychiatric and other nurse specialists providing mental health services under CHAMPUS with the American Nurses' Association, and for marriage and family therapists with the American Association of Marriage and Family Therapists. Each association has played a major role in designing credentialing guidelines for CHAMPUS certification, recruiting, and training its peer reviewers, and developing treatments reflecting professional evaluations and that not only are unique to the profession but also within generally accepted standards of care provided in the United States by other mental health professions. Furthermore, the five associations provide joint advisory assistance to CHAMPUS on an as-needed basis and will assist in developing joint data analysis research and educational plans. Efforts are also underway to consolidate peer review operations into one office. Throughout this conjoining, autonomous professional roles and functions will continue to be promoted.

Among the foci of these efforts is the ongoing refinement of review criteria and protocols, the development of pilot projects to monitor selected practices, and the expansion of routine reviews into specialized areas of practice.

Most likely, criteria development will involve greater use of objective rating scales (e.g., Global Assessment Scale, Role Function Scale) and research diagnostic criteria, such as those included in the DSM-III (American Psychiatric Association 1980), because third-party payers need to understand the indications for, and progress in, psychotherapy in the most specific and objective means possible. As previously mentioned, specialized peer review will continue to require attention. Reviewers with expertise in certain treatment modalities (e.g., hypnosis, biofeedback, psychoanalysis, child psychiatry, behavioral technology) or who also render care in selected treatment settings (e.g., outpatient brief dynamic psychotherapy, psychiatric partial hospitalization, residential treatment center services) need to be identified and matched with cases reflecting their special knowledge and skills. In addition, the efficacy and indications for direct peer review—where mutually consenting practitioner and reviewer meet face-to-face to discuss rendered care—need to be explored. Furthermore, the roles of psychiatric district branches or other mental health professional organizations operating their own peer review systems should also be evaluated.

The appropriate interventions of reviewers at prescribed review points merits examination as CHAMPUS and other third-party payers increase their volume of automated reviews. With the introduction of DRGs (diagnosis-related groups), claims review will allow focused reviews of selective providers, conducting certain procedures and at certain facilities. New financing systems will prompt the reevaluation of peer review since its very existence could be jeopardized with refinements in automated management. As a result, peer review outcomes must be measured and their effectiveness demonstrated, like other program elements. Furthermore, professional associations must actively market peer review and the effective performance of its reviewers, particularly in an increasingly competitive environment with the growth of private review organizations. CHAMPUS' special relationships with the APA and the

American Psychological Association will be tested and challenged by these many requirements and developments, particularly if economic considerations continue to gain ascendance in program management decisions. Thus, while much planning is geared toward future partnership, the essential unpredictability of the future will ultimately determine the survivability of peer review—at CHAMPUS and other third-party payers.

## Variables and Constants in Peer Review

There are many variables that could shape the future direction of CHAMPUS' peer review project and peer review in general. Although this chapter will not detail potential alternative health scenarios or consequences occurring in CHAMPUS and other health benefits programs, some general notations should be made about those variables. Certainly the national economy and the twin bears of recession and inflation are crucial dependent variables. If these phenomena continue, particularly in consort with growth in the health care industry and demand for health services, health care costs will undoubtedly continue to rise at rates that will soon outstrip available finances to pay for those services. Alternative responses to this scenario will include increasing revenues through taxation or cost-share for public programs, increased premiums for private programs, or even decreased benefits. Mental health practitioners should be most concerned about either situation because of third-party payers' historical trend of questioning mental health benefits during lean times. In addition, the alternatives would directly affect the circumstances and revenues under which psychotherapy is provided.

Costs will also drive third-party payers to explore and engage in prospective reimbursement arrangements such as health maintenance organizations and preferred provider organizations. While elements of peer review have been inimical to both of these alternative health delivery systems, the form and personality that peer review would take under these programs is uncertain. The potential for programs such as CHAMPUS and Medicare to shift operations toward use of vouchers is still very real. In such an arrangement, program administrative costs would be greatly reduced and quality assurance would be provided through a combination of competitive enticements made by health services vendors and through the threat of malpractice litigation. If such changes are not effected, third-party payers will undoubtedly have to turn to a combination of automation, highly delineated benefits monitored by professionally developed review criteria sets, and selective professional review. The portion of professional review actually performed by peers is a function of the availability of the reviewers for "on demand" reviews and the cost-benefits of the review. In this instance, the professionally determined quality of care issues will be increasingly subsumed by economic and management priorities.

The role of the professional associations—particularly national associations—in today's health care marketplace can only be speculated. However, it is apparent that the economically driven competition we are now witnessing will severely test the abilities of any professional association to recruit members and to dictate practice standards to members or nonmembers. I suspect that it is likely that professional review will continue because it has demonstrated its effectiveness in claims determinations, thus reinforcing cost containment. However, benefit programs like CHAMPUS will have to consider the available peer review services offered by such entities as PSROs at some time in the future. CHAMPUS may also consider requiring practitioners to submit completed peer review reports as a condition for reimbursement. Thus the shifting winds of future economic trends and health care costs will drive all of these determinations and will either lead to more highly constructed administrative systems of peer review or free market-oriented and decentralized review processes. Although this might signal foreboding for the current arrangement between CHAMPUS and national mental health professional organizations, it poses unique challenges for fresh approaches to peer review.

The constants in peer review should be reaffirmed at each turn in the planning for future peer review systems. First and foremost, peer review is review of peers by peers. Nonprofessionals and nonpeers cannot supplant peer review. Although some might consider this point parochial, experience with peer review has repeatedly shown that peer review is more specific, accountable, consistent, and effective than nonpeer professional review. Also, peer review systems must continually push to provide for as much local involvement as possible in review—particularly as spurs to spontaneous local professional peer review supervision. The more local practitioners become effective in monitoring their own and their peers' local practices and shaping them to conform with established profession-wide standards of care, the less third-party payers will need to be in the business of regulating the professional through imposition of peer review as a condition of reimbursement. Finally, peer review will continue to require profession-specific delineations of what evaluations and treatments are medically (psychologically) necessary and to require the highest possible controls to ensure confidentiality. These essential aspects of peer review are what make it a professional system, with all of the higher ethical requirements that only a profession can best represent and assure. The skill of the professions in demonstrating their ability to effect peer review as a means of assuring quality and cost-conscious care will ultimately determine its future. Success in this task will be measured by the continuing interest and support of third-party payers, such as CHAMPUS, in paying for the review and ensuring that it is a constant in their business.

## REFERENCES

American Psychiatric Association: Psychiatric Utilization Review: Principles and Objectives, 3rd ed. Washington, DC, American Psychiatric Association, 1975

American Psychiatric Association: Manual of Psychiatric Peer Review. Washington, DC, American Psychiatric Association, 1976

American Psychiatric Association: Diagnostic and Statistical Manual of Mental Disorders, 3rd ed. Washington, DC, American Psychiatric Association, 1980

Asher J: Assuring Quality Mental Health Services: The CHAMPUS Experience (DHHS Publication No. ADM 81-1099). Rockville, Maryland, Alcohol, Drug Abuse, and Mental Health Administration, 1981

Bent R: Multidimensional model for control of private information. Professional Psychology 13:27–33, 1982a

Bent R: The quality assurance process as a management method for psychology training programs. Professional Psychology 13:98–104, 1982b

Claiborn W: The problem of professional incompetence. Professional Psychology 13:153–158, 1982

Claiborn W, Stricker G: Professional standards review organizations, peer review and CHAMPUS. Professional psychology 10:631–639, 1979

Claiborn W, Biskin B, Friedman L: CHAMPUS and quality assurance. Professional Psychology 13:40–49, 1982a

Claiborn W, Stricker G, Bent R (eds): Peer review and quality assurance (special issue). Professional Psychology 13(1), 1982b

Cohen L: Peer review of psychodynamic psychotherapy: an experimental study of the APA/CHAMPUS program. Professional Psychology 12:776–784, 1981

Cohen L, Holstein C: Characteristics and attitudes of peer reviewers and providers in psychology. Professional Psychology 13:66–73, 1982a

Cohen L, Holstein C: Year of degree and psychologists' attitudes towards peer review. Professional Psychology 13:175–180, 1982b

Cohen L, Nelson D: Peer review of psychodynamic psychotherapy. Evaluation and the Health Professions 5:130–144, 1982

Cohen L, Oyster-Nelson C: Clinicians' evaluation of psychodynamic psychotherapy: experimental data on psychological peer review. J Consult Clin Psychol 49:583–589, 1981

Cohen L, Pizzirusso D: Document-based peer review of psychodynamic psychotherapy: experimental studies of the American Psychological Association/CHAMPUS program. Evaluation and the Health Professions (in press)

Department of Defense: Regulation 6010.8-R: Civilian Health and Medical Program of the Uniformed Services. Washington, DC, Department of Defense and Department of Health, Education, and Welfare, 10 January 1977

Deuschle J, Alvarez B, Logsdon D, Stahl W, Smith H: Physician performance in a prepaid health plan: results of the peer review program of the Health Insurance Plan of Greater New York. Med Care 20:127–142, 1982

Dorken H: CHAMPUS ten-state claim experience for mental disorders: fiscal year 1975. Am Psychol 9:697–710, 1977

Military Medical Benefits Act of 1966; Sec. 55, 10 U.S.C, 1966

Morton S: Peer review: a view from within. Professional Psychology 13:141–144, 1982

Offenkrantz W: Psychoanalytic peer review today. The American Psychoanalytic Association Newsletter 16:6, 8, 1982

Office of Civilian Health and Medical Program of the Uniformed Services: Manual for Inpatient and Outpatient Psychiatric Claims Review. Aurora, Colorado, Office of Civilian Health and Medical Program of the Uniformed Services, 1980a

Office of Civilian Health and Medical Program of the Uniformed Services: User's Guide for Psychiatric Reports for Care Under the CHAMPUS Program in Fiscal Year 1980. Aurora, Colorado, Office of Civilian Health and Medical Program of the Uniformed Services, 1980b

Office of Civilian Health and Medical Program of the Uniformed Services: CHAMPUS Chartbook of OCHAMPUS Statistics. Aurora, Colorado, Office of Civilian Health and Medical Program of the Uniformed Services, 1984

Penner N: The CHAMPUS issue. Journal of the National Association of Private Psychiatric Hospitals 6:17–24, 1975

Rodriguez A: Psychological and psychiatric peer review at CHAMPUS. Am Psychol 38:941–947, 1983

Rodriguez A: The Role of Third-Party Payers in Determining Future Health Care in the U.S. Unpublished manuscript, 1983

Rodriguez A: Peer review program sets trend in claims processing. Business and Health 1:21–25, 1984

Sharfstein S: Implications of Cost Benefit Research in Mental Health Settings. Unpublished paper presented at the Workshop on Cost Benefits, Washington, DC, 1982

Shueman S, Troy W: Education and peer review. Professional Psychology 13:58–65, 1982

Sinclair C, Frankel M: The effect of quality assurance activities on the quality of mental health services. QRB 8:4-9, 1982

Snipe J: CHAMPUS utilization review and quality assurance programs, in Health Decision Systems. Edited by Hinman EJ. Chicago, Year Book Medical Publishers, 1980

Stricker G: Criteria for insurance review of psychological services. Professional Psychology 10:118–122, 1974

Stricker G: Personality assessment and insurance reimbursement. J Pers Assess 42:317–318, 1978

Stricker G: Peer review of outpatient psychological services, in Evaluation of Quality of Care in Psychiatry. Edited by Awad AG, Durost HB, McCornick WO. Elmsford, NY, Pergamon Press, 1980

Stricker G: Current status of the CHAMPUS program. The Psychologist-Psychoanalyst 2:12–13, 1981

Stricker G: Peer Review: The CHAMPUS Program. Unpublished Paper presented at the meeting of the American Psychological Association Convention, Washington, DC, 1982

Stricker G: Peer review systems in psychology, in Professional Psychologists' Handbook. Edited by Sales DB. New York, Plenum Press (in press)

Stricker G, Cohen L: The APA/CHAMPUS peer review project: implications for research and practice. Manuscript submitted for publication, 1983

Stricker G, Sechrest L: The role of research in criteria construction. Professional Psychology 13:19–22, 1982

Stricker G, Claiborn W, Bent R: Peer review: an overview. Professional Psychology 13:5–8, 1982

U.S. Senate, 93rd Congress: Defense Department's CHAMPUS Program (hearings before the permanent Subcommittee on Investigations of the Committee on Government Operations, Parts 1 and 2, 23–26 July 1974). Washington, DC, U.S. Government Printing Office, 1974

Willens J, DeLeon P: Political aspects of peer review. Professional Psychology 13-27–33, 1982

Williamson J (ed): Teaching Quality Assurance and Cost Containment in Health Care: A Faculty Guide. San Francisco, Jossey-Bass, 1982

Williamson J, Hudson J, Nevons M: Principles of Quality Assurance and Cost Containment in Health Care: A Guide for Medical Students, Residents and Other Health Professionals. San Francisco, Jossey-Bass, 1982

Wooden K: Weeping in the Playtime of Others: America's Incarcerated Children. New York, McGraw-Hill, 1976

Young, H: Alternatives in mental health care and criteria for quality assurance. Professional Psychology 13:91–97, 1982

Zaro J, Kilburg R: The role of APA in the development of quality assurance in psychological practice. Professional Psychology 12:112–118, 1982

# 8

# A Peer Review Primer

*Ronald S. Mintz, M.D.*

# A Peer Review Primer

The apprentice system of training medical students, which has existed since the earliest days of medical history, can be considered an early example of medical peer review. This system has continued in modern medical training, both at the bedside and in presentations before one's peers (and superiors) in grand rounds and in various aspects of internship and residency training. Written and performance tests required for state licensure or other certification (such as diplomate of a medical speciality board) may also be seen as examples of review by one's peers. Procedures leading to hospital staff privileges, promotion in rank on the faculty of a medical school, or elevation to fellow status in a national medical organization may also involve peer review. On a more informal level, each of us may perform private peer review when we consider referring a patient to a medical colleague.

Hospital staff committees have for some years established various standards of medical practice to which the medical activities of their peers may be compared. Some of these standards consist of codified parameters of locally or nationally acceptable medical care. Members of the hospital medical staff whose activities and practices reflect a pattern that deviates from such established standards may be reviewed by an appropriate hospital committee of their peers.

141

Public and private legal proceedings involving expert medical testimony regarding community standards of medical practice constitute another example of peer review.

It is only during the last decade, however, that peer review has taken on a more defined and explicit meaning. This has come about due to the requirements of federal law, which mandate that certain medical activities of all physicians treating Medicare patient be subjected to peer review (Social Security Amendments of 1972). Thus a single law introduced medical peer review into almost every hospital in the nation.

## BASIC DEFINITIONS

### Inpatient Hospital Utilization Review

First-level review consists of various clerical tasks, such as reviewing header information for completeness, verifying the current eligibility of the patient for health benefits under a given program, and reviewing demographic data for obvious contradictions (e.g., when the birth date does not correspond to the age that has been listed).

Second-level review consists of the review of the medical reasonableness and necessity for hospital admission, the medical appropriateness of the treatment plan and services rendered, the timeliness and appropriateness of discharge and postdischarge plans, and other relevant aspects of medical and paramedical services. Second-level review is carried out by a medically knowledgeable individual who is *not* a peer of the treating physician. Most frequently, the second-level review is conducted by a nurse.

In many (but not all) settings, a nonphysician carrying out second-level review has the authority to approve reviewed procedures but must consult a physician when they do not conform to screening criteria.

The term *peer* may be broadly defined, such as "any physician reviewing another physician's treatment records." Sometimes the term is defined more narrowly, such as "a physician who is a psychiatrist and a psychoanalyst," or "a board-certified child psychiatrist reviewing the psychiatric inpatient hospital treatment of a child."

On occasion, fourth-level review is encountered. It refers to the review of a sample of peer review decisions carried out by a review committee or organization. An example would be the periodic review by a Professional Standards Review Organization (PSRO) of sample peer reviews carried out by a hospital utilization review committee.

Second- or third-level review may be concurrent (carried out while the patient is still in the hospital) or retrospective (carried out after the patient has been discharged from the hospital). In addition, preadmission certification is an example of a prospective review; it is conducted prior to the delivery of health services.

First-, second- and third-level reviews are usually document-based since they rely on the patient's medical records for information. However, peer review could also be conducted by interviewing the patient or the treating physician to assess the status or outcome of the treatment episode.

Second- or third-level utilization review is implemented for a variety of purposes, such as to ensure quality of care, to verify that the most appropriate and cost-effective treatment plan is being followed, to comply with federal Medicare or Medicaid requirements, or to assist third-party payers in making payment decisions for rendered services.

## Outpatient Hospital or Outpatient Office Utilization Review

Similar reviews of medical records may be carried out with respect to outpatient hospital, home, or office medical diagnostic and treatment services. Often the review is based on a narrative clinical summary or information requested on a mental illness treatment form prepared by the treating physician.

## Implicit Assumptions

Peer review is generally carried out using specified or implicit assumptions.

## Documentation

The treating physician must document in the medical record conclusions as well as information supporting the findings. To promote accurate and equitable reviews, it is important for all relevant information to be included in narrative summaries or treatment reports.

## Level of Care

Third-party payers and government benefit programs advocate treatment of the patient at the lowest level of care consistent with safety and efficacy. Therefore, the patient should not be hospitalized if treatment can be safely and effectively performed on an outpatient basis.

## Timeliness

Diagnostic procedures, treatment, and consultations should be ordered and carried out in a timely manner. A critical area relating to timeliness is discharge planning, which should be initiated at or near the time of admission.

## Effective Treatment

Treatment known to be effective for the patient's medical condition should be utilized, unless a clear and medically acceptable explanation is entered in the medical records.

# UTILIZATION AND PEER REVIEW CRITERIA

Utilization and peer review may be conducted with any one of two principal sets of criteria:

## Implicit Criteria

Very often the criterion utilized is the informed medical judgment of the reviewer. It is assumed, for example, that a physician who has removed a large number of gall bladders is capable of appropriately evaluating the medical reasonableness and necessity of the operative treatment for patients with this disease.

## Explicit Criteria

Sometimes established criteria are utilized that have been derived from a survey or consensus regarding customary treatment in the community. Community may be defined as a small geographic area, such as a city, or a larger geo-

A Peer Review Primer

graphic locality, such as a state. Another type of explicit criteria represents the combined judgment of knowledgeable persons in the medical field (such as providers and third-party payers) regarding minimal acceptable treatment standards. Such standards may or may not bear any close relationship to actual current community standards.

Standards may be developed by a variety of groups, such as a hospital peer review committee, a PSRO medical criteria committee, a medical advisory board to an insurance company, the U.S. Public Health Service, a county or state medical society, a professional association such as the American Psychiatric Association (APA), a governmental agency such as the Health Care Financing Administration of the Department of Health and Human Services, or a committee of individuals who are generally accepted in the medical community as experts regarding a given subject of medical practice.

## Specificity

Criteria vary widely in their degree of operational specificity. The examples of criteria shown in Table 1 are incomplete, but are presented as illustrative of varying degrees of criteria specificity.

**Table 1.** Justification for Admission to Inpatient Alcoholism Rehabilitation Treatment

*Non-specific*
1. Excessive use of alcohol

*Intermediate*
1. Meets DSM-III (American Psychiatric Association 1980) criteria for diagnosis of alcohol dependence
2. Has a reasonable likelihood of significant improvement in response to rehabilitation treatment, based on a documented evaluation of motivation, life support systems, and current life situation.

*Specific*
1. Meets DSM-III criteria for diagnosis of alcohol dependence
2. Has a concomitant acute illness requiring hospital level of care, or
3. Has failed in an outpatient alcoholism rehabilitation program within the past nine months after attending at least three full weeks. The program must have been specifically designed to treat chronic alcoholics; provided group therapy, educational services, and individual counseling; and kept written treatment records.

## Criteria Sets

Criteria may be diagnosis specific. The model screening criteria sets contained in the *Manual of Psychiatric Peer Review* (American Psychiatric Association 1981) are examples of diagnosis-specific criteria sets.

Criteria sets that are not diagnosis specific have been developed. For example, the Task Force on Insurance Code Project ranks patient illness episodes by severity (American Psychiatric Association 1982). Certain psychiatric diagnoses are usually, but not always, related to specific degrees of severity. Some PSROs have developed criteria sets that relate the need for treatment (regardless of diagnosis) to severity of illness and intensity of services.

## Screening versus Definitive Criteria

Review criteria are frequently developed in such a manner as to include some 70 to 95 percent of all acceptable cases. Such criteria constitute "screening" criteria. Cases not meeting these criteria are referred for physician peer review. Peer reviewers often approve cases as medically reasonable and necessary even though they do not meet the customary screening criteria. In these instances, special circumstances that render the hospitalization medically appropriate may be present.

*Example:* A stable, nonsuicidal depressed patient may not generally require an acute hospitalization for initiation of treatment with a tricyclic antidepressant medication. However, if the patient has a severe cardiac dysfunction, it may be quite appropriate to hospitalize the patient initially to ensure continuous skilled nursing observation.

*Example:* The usual maximum length of stay for combined alcohol detoxification and rehabilitation treatment under Medicare is 21 days. If a significant breakthrough in the patient's capacity for honest self-confrontation occurs on the 20th day of hospitalization, it may be medically appropriate to retain the patient in the hospital for several additional days to consolidate this significant change.

From the standpoint of providing optimal quality of medical care, it is desirable that, wherever possible, third-party payers and providers recognize that the criteria were developed for screening purposes only. This leaves room for medical peer review to assess the presence or absence of special circumstances that affect the medical reasonableness and necessity of treatment being rendered at the given level of care.

## A Model Peer Review Program

A brief description is included here of the PSRO model of concurrent hospital peer review. The APA's peer review program is described in detail elsewhere in this volume.

## Acute versus Rehabilitation Treatment Services

Acute care consists of evaluation or treatment of a patient for medical conditions of a brief duration. In each case, the medical necessity of the hospital admission must be documented, as well as the medical necessity for continuing stay. In second- and third-level utilization review, the approved length of stay also depends on the documented medical necessity.

Rehabilitation treatment consists of intensive (and usually multidisciplinary) treatment of a patient for a chronic condition. The rehabilitation program must conform to explicit standards pertaining to staffing patterns, admission requirements, and regular patient-care conferences. Furthermore, rehabilitation programs often have general treatment ideologies with usual lengths of stay. In some programs, the maximum length of stay is immutable; in others, the usual maximum length of stay may be exceeded for documented medical need. Appropriate admissions must document that the patient met certain criteria involving symptomatology, prior treatment efforts, and prognosis. For example, for admission to a chronic pain rehabilitation program, the patient must demonstrate: (1) existence of a chronic pain condition; (2) that the usual methods for treatment of the condition were tried without significant success; (3) existence of a significant functional limitation as a consequence of the chronic pain condition; and (4) reasonable expectation of improvement based on such factors as motivation and family support.

## DIAGNOSIS-RELATED GROUPS
## AND PEER REVIEW

For hospital fiscal years beginning on or after 1 October 1983, each hospital in the United States treating Medicare patients came under a new system of reimbursement from the federal government. This new system is called the Diagnosis-Related Groups—Prospective Payment System (DRG—PPS). Under the prior system of reimbursement, hospitals were paid for allowable charges. Thus each additional day of a patient's hospital stay generated additional money for the hospital. (Some restrictions were imposed by the 1972 Social Security Amendments and the Tax Equity and Fiscal Responsibility Act of 1982.) Under the new DRG—PPS system, the 11,000 diagnoses of the ICD-9-CM (Commission on Professional and Hospital Activities 1979) have been categorized by researchers at Yale University into 23 major diagnostic categories (MDCs) and further divided into 467 basic categories of DRGs. This categorization is based on such data elements as the principal diagnosis, complications and comorbidity conditions, principal diagnostic and operative procedures, age, and discharge destination. It is intended that the diagnostic conditions in each DRG utilize roughly the same intensity of hospital resources. A reimbursement weight has been assigned to each DRG. The hospital is paid the same dollar amount for a patient whose stay is categorized in a given DRG whether the patient is in the hospital for 1 day or for 20 days.

Thus the DRG—PPS is a prospective pricing system, with marked implications for hospital financial solvency and for issues of peer review. Under the old system, peer review activities attempted to reduce unnecessary hospital days so as to reduce the government's Medicare health care costs. Under the new system it is the hospital that is at risk for unnecessary or uneconomical expenditures.

Psychiatric hospitals and distinct psychiatric wards in general hospitals are temporarily exempted from the DRG—PPS system and will continue under the prior system of cost-based reimbursement. However, the secretary of the Department of Health and Human Services must report to Congress in 1985 regarding the feasibility of including psychiatric hospitals and psychiatric wards of general hospitals in the DRG system. (The secretary also had to report to Congress in 1984 regarding the feasibility of including payment for the physician's professional services in the DRG payment.)

In New Jersey, the hospitals are reimbursed for all services (public or private), including psychiatric services, according to a DRG system. The New Jersey DRG system has features that make it financially less stringent than the Medicare DRG–PPS system. In several states, private health insurance plans such as Blue Cross have already begun to reimburse hospitals, including psychiatric hospitals, using DRG. This approach to hospital reimbursement is likely to expand.

Under a DRG system, peer review functions must focus on a number of issues relating to quality of care. Was the patient retained in the hospital sufficiently long to receive appropriate care of the medical condition? Did the patient receive all the diagnostic services that were appropriate?

## SOME FINAL COMMENTS

We live in an age in which increased accountability is a requirement. Peer review provides the opportunity for reducing unnecessary medical costs and for ensuring an acceptable level of quality of medical care. Various models of peer review may be devised to fit particular circumstances or regulations. In the next few years an increasing percentage of hospital admissions, including admissions for the treatment of psychiatric illnesses, are likely to be evaluated through concurrent peer review. Physicians must be involved in the establishment of peer review criteria, analysis of data, and general administration and conduct of peer review programs. Otherwise, the fundamental criterion of medical necessity of each individual case may be supplanted by a schedule of statistical averages.

## REFERENCES

American Psychiatric Association: Diagnostic and Statistical Manual of Mental Disorders, 3rd ed. Washington, DC, American Psychiatric Association, 1980

American Psychiatric Association: Manual of Psychiatric Peer Review. Washington, DC, American Psychiatric Association, 1981

American Psychiatric Association and the Health Insurance Association of America: Psychiatric Coding System for Insurance Claims Reporting. Washington, DC, American Psychiatric Association, 1982

Commission on Professional and Hospital Activities: The International Classification of Diseases, 9th ed. Ann Arbor, Michigan, Edwards Brothers, 1979

Social Security Amendments of 1972, PL 92-603, Part 6, Title XI, 1972

# 9

# Residential Treatment Facilities and Their Place in the Mental Health Care Delivery System

*Charles F. Marsh, M.D.*
*Joseph R. Mawhinney, M.D.*
*Henry A. Davis, M.D.*
*Gary L. Shepherd, M.D.*

# Residential Treatment Facilities and Their Place in the Mental Health Care Delivery System

## TOWARDS AN INTEGRATED MODEL

Over the last 20 years many residential treatment centers have developed. According to a National Institute of Mental Health (NIMH) staffing survey done in 1974, there were 340 such facilities in the United States. Although numerous different treatments have been utilized over the past 10 to 15 years, two particular models have become prominent. The first model, which began in the 1950s, places heavy emphasis on "individually centered treatment," involving

This effort was sponsored and requested by OCHAMPUS under contract no. MDA-90683-C-002. This endeavor was directed by Gary L. Shepherd, M.D., and significant input and editing were done by the entire Mental Health Treatment Committee of the San Diego Psychiatric Society. It was completed in November 1981.

**Editor's Note:** This chapter has been included in this book because residential treatment of adolescents was a critical area at the beginning of the development of our current peer review process and required an intense assessment to correct many perceived difficulties in this particular treatment setting. It continues to be a critical area for psychiatry. This section provides a detailed look at a segment of our system of service delivery which illustrates the way in which peer review can be instrumental in providing a third-party assurance that medically necessary and appropriate care has been provided. This chapter summarizes the experiences of the San Diego Psychiatric Society.

one-to-one therapeutic relationships. Individual psychotherapy is conducted almost as though it were virtually
isolated from the child's enviroment. Environmental experiences are seen as important but the main thrust of treatment revolves around the individual therapy.

The second model, whose roots developed in the early
1960s, is more of an environmental model. In this approach, summation of all environmental experiences is seen
as the actual treatment. The experience of living outside of
the home and in a more structured setting, being exposed
to rules and limits, and the opportunity to facilitate identification with better adult role models all play a part in the
treatment process. Living with peers in a group setting is
also part of this model, and the totality of the above-mentioned experiences are said to provide a "corrective living
experience" for the child. This basic approach relies on
learning theory; individual therapy is not an integral part of
this program. However, the "Re-Ed" (re-education) programs do rely on individual therapy.

The mental health care delivery system is complex and
divergent. It includes such services as private practice, state
mental health programs, community mental health clinics,
health maintenance organizations, and hospital programs.
Residential treatment is just one of many treatment
modalities on the continuum from outpatient services to
hospital treatment. Other alternative treatment modalities
include partial day treatment, regular and specialized foster
homes, therapeutic group homes, and "satellite" foster
homes (as hospital extensions). Satellite foster homes refer
to specialized long-term foster homes for severely disturbed
children, staffed by specially trained "house parents" with
mental health professional support and psychiatric hospital
back-up.

Figure 1 compares these treatment modalities and how
they relate to each other with regard to restrictiveness of
environment and comprehensiveness. In this particular
context, outpatient treatment is assumed to be the least
restrictive form of treatment and inpatient hospital treatment is assumed to be the most restrictive and intensive
form of treatment. For simplicity in this chapter, intensity is
assumed to increase with comprehensiveness. (This is generally true except in the case of intensive outpatient therapy.)

**Figure 1.** Comparison of various treatment modalities in relation to restrictiveness of environment and comprehensiveness of treatment.

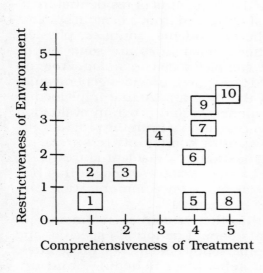

1. Patient living at home with outpatient treatment
2. Regular foster home.
3. Incentive foster home.
4. Therapeutic group home.
5. Partial day treatment.
6. Satellite foster home (as part of hospital extension).
7. Residential treatment center.
8. Partial hospitalization.
9. Long-term hospital care.
10. Short-term hospital care.

It must be noted that in any given community, the spectrum of services is dependant on a variety of social, political, and financial factors. Furthermore, coordination between the health care financing and health care delivery system is often lacking. Similarly, changes in the reimbursement system can cause disruptive consequences for the delivery system.

It is my contention that the current overutilization of hospital services and the relative lack of less restrictive and less comprehensive forms of treatment such as residential treatment, group homes, and day treatment are a disservice to the patients and a squandering of the limited mental health financial resources.

## PROGRAM AND TREATMENT

The therapeutic impact of residential treatment relates to the total experience of the child or adolescent in treatment.

For residential treatment to be effective, there must be a coordination and integration of multiple modalities into both a general treatment plan (program-wide) and an individual treatment plan.

The many interrelated components of residential treatment can perhaps be best described from a general systems perspective. Staff members, residents, routines, physical environment, and treatment modalities are some of the elements involved in this complex social organism. Program philosophy, which should be explicit, provides general guidance in development of the program. Actual implementation, integration of components, and program evaluation depend on effective communication within the program elements and externally to existing community resources.

The lines of communication in a residential treatment facility could be said to be the nervous system of this biosocial organism. A special focus on communication processes and their content is essential.

Communication within the residential treatment center's program components should be formal, specific, and enunciated in program philosophy statements, procedures, policies, routines, and schedules. Scheduled and unscheduled meetings should address community–staff, staff–resident, resident–staff, and resident–resident communication processes. Some techniques employed in residential treatment facilities include community meetings, one-to-one (staff–resident) and three-way (resident–staff–resident) conferences, and the use of the house log to enter comments and concerns more anonymously if desired.

A typical example of the effort to facilitate staff–staff communication are staff meetings that deal not only with general and individual treatment plans of the residents but also with the staff–group process. Issues addressed in this latter type of meeting may include:

1. Role definition
2. Leadership hierarchy
3. Countertransference issues
4. Therapeutic blindspots
5. Clarification of institutional policies and procedures
6. Program development issues
7. Communication patterns and problems

Crucial to treatment effectiveness is the integration of a full range of treatment modalities into the general and specific treatment plans of the residents. Typical modalities offered within the residential treatment facility would be:

1. Milieu treatment
2. Group therapy
3. Family therapy or family-oriented therapy
4. Individual therapy
5. Behavior modification principles and techniques
6. Psychopharmacology
7. Neuromedical evaluation and treatment
8. Sensory-motor therapy
9. Occupational therapy
10. Recreational therapy
11. Art therapy
12. Music, dance, movement therapy
13. Educational programs with special education components
14. Speech and language assessment and therapy
15. Vocational assessment, planning, and training

Communication between the residential treatment facility and the community system of direct and indirect services, as well as the political and policy-making agencies of the community, is essential for appropriate program planning and responsiveness to the needs of the community. Organized communication with other residential treatment facilities allows sharing of ideas, problems, and conflicts, as well as providing the opportunity for a significant voice in the political dialogue of the community.

The course of residential treatment may be described in five distinct phases for each individual resident. Program planning should relate to the special aspects of these phases.

## Intake Phase

Prior to admission, a thorough evaluation of the applicant should be completed. The evaluation should include (but not be limited to):

- History of past treatment,
- Developmental and psychosocial history,
- Neuro-medical history
- Psychological testing, and
- Educational evaluations and family assessment (in addition to current psychiatric evaluation indicating the level of functional impairment).

Clear indications of the need for residential treatment also should be provided, as well as diagnosis, prognosis, and projected length of stay.

The intake should involve a team of mental health professionals including a psychiatrist, psychologist, social worker, primary counselor (or mental health worker), program director, and others as indicated. Specific guidelines and criteria (inclusive and exclusive) for admission should be formulated by the residential treatment facility.

### Initial Treatment Phase

A settling-in period, often described as the honeymoon, normally lasts 1 to 2 months but may last 4 to 5 months. On rare occasions, the honeymoon may extend to as much as 8 to 10 months. This phase actually begins with the acceptance of the applicant into the program. A supportive and, if possible, stepwise transition from the previous residence into the facility is helpful in engaging the patient in the treatment process.

During the initial treatment phase, the resident may not show characteristic, symptomatic behavior. The task of integrating into the residential treatment facility community or "family" dominates this phase (e.g., assignment of primary staff counselor, assignment of residential big brother or sister, limiting family contacts). All of these serve to integrate the resident within the program. Relaxation of defenses used by the resident to cope with the strange, new environment and manifestation of preadmission symptomatic behavior marks the end of this phase.

### Middle Phase of Treatment

During this middle phase, the resident presents characteristic behavioral and interactional patterns including transferences and defenses, as well as ego strengths and ego deficits. Therapeutic change due to corrective life experiences (guided by ongoing evaluation and development of the treatment plan) is the primary goal of this phase. When appropriate, family involvement in the treatment plan is increased. Duration of this middle phase of treatment may range from a few months to 1 year. In a few cases involving severe but correctable ego deficits, duration of the middle phase of treatment may be as long as 2 or 3 years.

**Termination Phase of Treatment**

Although it could be rightfully said that termination is an issue from the time of admission (with prediction of an approximate length of stay), selection of a specific approximate discharge date results in a special focus on termination. Temporary regressions to earlier dysfunctional patterns often occur, allowing a final working through with special attention to issues of separation, loss, and reintegration into the family or community.

This may be a stormy period for many patients and their families. Duration of this phase is highly variable; generally 2 to 4 months is adequate to deal with and work through issues relating to termination and anticipation of the future. In some cases, however, as much as 6 to 8 months may be necessary. Some ego-deficient individuals (e.g., those with borderline personality organizations or schizophrenia) may experience multiple severe regressions requiring a year or more to complete this stage sufficiently to make a successful postdischarge adaptation.

**Aftercare and Follow-up**

Ongoing involvement and support during the transitional period into the community or other treatment setting is essential for successful implementation of the discharge plan. Return visitation or contact with the residential treatment facility after discharge should be structured and individualized according to the treatment plan to minimize regression while at the same time providing support and continuity where possible.

Although lengths of stay may be widely varied due to severity of pathology as well as social system factors, the average length of stay is 1 to 2 years. On rare occasions as much as 3 to 4 years may be necessary to allow successful termination and transition to a less restrictive environment.

Presently existing follow-up studies support the positive impact of residential treatment facility programs, but methodological problems such as inadequate criteria for admission, diagnosis, treatment, and follow-up render the results imprecise and of limited value. Nonetheless, follow-up evaluations and, where possible, formal research should be encouraged to provide feedback for program development and further refinement of research methodology. Funding of valid and reliable evaluation methods and research in this area should be a priority of private insurers, foundations, and government agencies.

## STAFFING

The backbone of any residential treatment facility is the staff. Facilities differ tremendously in this area. Psychiatry, psychology, and social work have traditionally played major roles in the staffing of residential facilities. Over the last decade, recreational, occupational, music, and art therapists have also established themselves as important members of the treatment team. In most facilities, the largest percentage of staff are mental health workers. Some facilities are very traditional and the major therapeutic work is performed by psychiatrists, psychologists, and social workers. In these centers, the mental health worker is a primary role model and a limit setter. Other facilities use other mental health workers such as occupational or recreational therapists in addition to psychiatrists, psychologists, and social workers, and give them major responsibilities for treatment.

In our opinion, the ideal model is one in which psychiatrists, psychologists and social workers play prominent roles because they have the most comprehensive clinical training. Individual therapy should be at least weekly and should be conducted by a therapist from one of these three licensed disciplines. Occupational and recreational therapy should be available to all residents. Music and art therapy should be provided on an individual or group basis, when appropriate. Mental health workers would be involved in setting limits and role modeling, but would also be trained and supervised by the professional staff to participate in group therapy, family therapy, psychodrama, and behavior modification. Clarity in role definition and a strong commitment to training and staff development all but ensure a better program. Comprehensive psychological testing and neuropsychological testing performed by a licensed clinical psychologist is an absolute necessity. The testing and assessment specialist may also be the best person to organize the staff development program. A licensed social worker experienced in developmental family therapy and the aftercare program is vital. A registered nurse or licensed practical nurse should be hired at least part time to organize general medical treatment with a consulting board-certified pediatrician.

A psychiatrist who has experience or training in the evaluation and treatment of children or adolescents should be an integral part of the staff. In this capacity, the psychiatrist should be involved in patient-centered, staff-centered, and program-centered consultations. The psychiatrist may also function as psychotherapist and as staff in-service trainer.

Every effort should be made to provide appropriate educational services to meet specialized needs of this patient population. The current trend is for provision of educational services by the public school system with staffing by a teacher with special education training. Speech, hearing, and language evaluation and therapy by qualified professionals should be available. In addition, vocational counseling and coordination of vocational training should be provided.

The ratio of staff to residents is very important. A ratio of one staff member for every three residents is ideal. The ratio will be affected by budgetary, administrative, and clinical factors. A patient population of more severely disturbed adolescents will require a higher staff-to-patient ratio.

## INDICATIONS FOR ADMISSION INTO RESIDENTIAL TREATMENT

Residential treatment is usually seen as one form of treatment for severely emotionally disturbed children and adolescents who do not need hospitalization but whose treatment requires a structured, comprehensive program, not possible in an outpatient or day treatment approach. This issue is complicated by the lack of a clear and widely accepted definition of severe emotional disturbance in children. In many cases, residential treatment is the treatment of choice, but in other cases it is the best treatment because other more appropriate treatments are not readily available. The majority of children exhibit behavior disorders, borderline personality disorders, psychotic disorders, and substance abuse. Common symptomatic problems of the patients in residential treatment may include stealing, truancy, running away, fire setting, learning difficulties, destructive behavior, and drug abuse. Subjective symptoms of confusion, depression, poor reality testing, and impaired judgment are common. The causes of the above-mentioned symptomatic picture are multiple and varied.

Much time should be devoted to the intake and pre-placement evaluation to assess the severity of the patient's psychopathology, the need for a residential treatment facility environment, and the ability of the patient to benefit from residential treatment. It should be determined that residential treatment is the most appropriate and least restrictive alternative available for the treatment of the patient's psychopathology.

Indications for admission to a residential treatment center include:

1. A patient manifesting a degree of psychopathology or functional impairment that would prevent successful outpatient treatment, but would not require the intensity and structure of a psychiatric hospital.
2. A patient who is in need of a highly specialized environment that provides structure, stability, restrictiveness, and protectiveness.
3. The absence of more appropriate and less restrictive or less intensive treatment alternatives.
4. A patient with the ability to benefit from a residential treatment center, possessing such favorable indicators as relatively intact ego function, subjective experience of distress, and motivation for change.
5. A patient whose family is involved and committed to the treatment process and lives in close proximity to the residential treatment facility.

In addition to the above indications for admission, other factors to consider include:

1. The personal needs of the applicant and the ability of the program to meet these needs (i.e., dietary, medical, cultural, educational, religious, or spiritual).
2. Specific developmental needs of the applicant (e.g., separate programming is necessary for preschool, preadolescent, and adolescent populations).
3. The needs of the milieu (e.g., population balance, cohesion, manageability).
4. Skills of the staff in dealing with special areas (e.g., developmental disabilities, autism, severe psychosis).
5. Evaluation of the preplacement visit or visits of the applicant and the family.
6. Recommendation of appropriate alternatives if admission is not indicated.

Some unfavorable indications for admission into residential treatment include:

1. Existence of very severe character pathology, particularly antisocial or schizoid type.
2. Florid psychotic symptomatology.
3. Long history of violently aggressive behavior, including assaultiveness.
4. Failure of previous residential treatment.
5. Referrals from distant county agencies with whom there is no close cooperation.
6. Family or relatives not readily available for evaluation and treatment (although in some cases this separation and lack of involvement may be a positive factor).
7. Resistance of the family and the patient to therapeutic change.

Although it is assumed by many that mentally retarded children do not benefit from residential treatment, this has not been borne out by the authors' experiences, nor by the literature. Specialized treatment techniques are required, however, for the more severely impaired. These techniques may be utilized in special "tracks" within a residential treatment facility or utilized comprehensively in specialized residential treatment facilities.

The decision-making process in the admission of a child or adolescent to a residential treatment facility is extremely complex and demanding. A better understanding of residential treatment as one specific modality within the broader continuum of treatment modalities would perhaps help prevent inappropriate utilization. Hopefully, a clearer delineation of indications and contraindications for admission will assist in achieving this goal. However, it is important to recognize that none of the factors cited above are absolute and each case should be evaluated on an individual basis with all factors taken into consideration. A diagnosis of character disorder, for example, is not an absolute contraindication for admission because certain characterologically impaired children and adolescents can receive considerable benefit from this form of treatment. However, diagnoses of antisocial or schizoid character disorders do have a less favorable prognosis, particularly in the absence of favorable support systems.

## REVIEW CRITERIA

Periodic review of treatment plans with regard to attainment of goals, endpoints, and changes in clinical status is an integral part of good treatment. Treatment plans should be written with attention to presenting problems, short- and long-term goals, specific treatment methods planned to accomplish each goal, and identification of the person or persons responsible for carrying out the treatment method. A specific statement should be made as to the role of individual and family treatment in the overall treatment plan.

In the 2 weeks following admission, a detailed treatment plan and clinical evaluation should be developed by the interdisciplinary team and submitted to the utilization review committee with its identified target problems, goals, and methods. For purposes of tracking, three or four major problem areas that are significant with regard to return to the community may be identified. The data base for this report will be primarily obtained from the intake phase and will necessarily be modified during the course of treatment. Formal written review of the clinical status and treatment plan of the child or adolescent (psychiatric review) should be made at intervals no greater than 6 months and more

**Figure 2.**  Sample Format for Formal Psychiatric Review

Psychiatric Review

| | |
|---|---|
| Name: | Diagnostic Impression |
| BD:(birth date) | |
| Adm. (admission) Date: | Medication |
| Date of report: | |

---

A. *Treatment Plan*—(Sample format)

   *Problem*   (Statement of the presenting problem and underlying dynamics or causes)

   *Goals*                    *Methods*  (specific treatment methods and who is responsible)

      *Short-term*

      *Long-term*

   *Progress*  (Brief statement of status of goals in relation to last psychiatric review; evaluate degree of success, effectiveness of treatment methods employed, appropriateness of goal, and recommendations for its continuation or change)

B. *Clinical Status Report*
    (Covers other major areas of interest in addition to the treatment plan)

    The 15 points of this section are detailed in the example. For review purposes, each point should be addressed. Behavioral and other information should be used to show progress.

frequently as requested by reviewers. These reports should track previously identified problems and goals and also include current additions, deletions, and modifications of the treatment plan. These major reviews should document involvement by the multidisciplinary team, including the psychiatric consultant.

Specific aftercare and follow-up plans should be included in the reviews, with goals and methods signed off by responsible staff within 6 months after discharge.

An interim residential treatment facility review should be accomplished by the interdisciplinary team every 90 days, the summary of which should be available in a clinical record for each resident. These reports should reflect treatment plans, changes, progress, success or failure in achieving goals, and a discussion where indicated. In addition, continued indications for residential treatment should be cited. Weekly or bimonthly treatment team meetings should be recorded and participants listed.

Figure 2 shows a sample format for the formal written review referred to above, including a goal-oriented treatment plan and clinical status report, as used in the case report that follows.

## Case Example

### Psychiatric Review

Name: John Thompson            Diagnostic Impression
BD: 9/22/64
Adm. Date: 10/12/79                1. Episodic Dyscontrol
Date of report: 4/20/80            2. Borderline
                                      Personality

                                   Medication:
                                      Haldol 2 mg b.i.d.

---

A. *Treatment Plan*
   *Problem #1*
      Assaultive behavior
         When under stress, particularly that associated with perceived rejection, John reacts with intense rage, attacking anyone whom he perceives as an enemy. Reality testing at these times is poor.

   *Goals*                          *Methods*

      *Short-term*
      1. Prevent injury to       1. Intervene at earliest pos-
         others                      sible moment (All staff)
      2. Decrease frequency    1. Psychotropic medications
         and intensity of as-      (M. Smith, M.D.)
         saultive behavior

2. Help John to anticipate reaction and develop conscious controls through individual and group therapy (M. Smith, M.D., individual therapist; J. Jones, M.A. and T. Jackson, M.H.W., group therapists)

3. Improve reality testing

1. Psychotropic medications (M. Smith, M.D.)

2. Provide reality feedback regarding relationships and situations that might be interpreted by him as rejection or separation from dependency object (All staff)

*Long-term*
1. Develop effective aggressive impulse control

1. Develop improved controls through anticipation and intervention (All staff)

2. Find socially acceptable means to express aggressive feelings (e.g., sports, punching bag, verbalization) (All staff)

3. Work through underlying conflict related to separation and individuation in individual and family therapy. (M. Smith, M.D., individual therapist; J. James, M.A. and M. White, M.H.W., family therapists)

4. Family therapy deferred at this time (see below)

<table>
<tr>
<td>2. Develop ability to tolerate criticism from or withdrawal or separation by dependency figure</td>
<td>1. Individual and family therapy to work through separations and individuation issues<br><br>2. Improve self-esteem by building on positive skills (e.g., academic, sports, writing, school, activities and recreation) (All staff)</td>
</tr>
</table>

*Progress*

There has been one incidence of assaultive behavior in the first 6 months of treatment compared to three such episodes in the 6 months prior to admission. This episode was serious in that he attacked a staff member with the apparent intention of doing bodily harm and he required four male staff to restrain him. During this period he perceived all others as hostile to him and as "keeping him from his mother." He recovered within 2 hours and exhibited remorse and feelings of guilt for his behavior. It is felt that the patient is just ending the initial treatment phase and that the above episode represents his characteristic pattern of conflicted dependency relationships with episodic psychotic regression under appropriate stress. To reduce and possibly to prevent further such episodes, Haldol 2 mg b.i.d. has been prescribed.

It is anticipated that more frequent outbursts will be seen in coming months and that with treatment, expression of aggressive affect will be increasingly displaced or sublimated (e.g., destruction of property; verbal abuse; physical exercise such as weights, punching bag, contact sports, noncontact sports; verbal discussion; creative activity). There is some danger of self-destructive or even overt suicidal behavior during early phases of this process.

Current goals should be continued. Family therapy is not yet appropriate due to John's intense and potentially dangerous reactions, as well as his lack of any insight or conscious anticipation of the conflict.

John continues to need the structure and intensity of treatment provided by residential treatment. Hospital back-up is available for short-term treatment of severe regression endangering himself or others.

B. *Clinical Status Report*

   1. Medical/Neurological: Current status, changes since last report, diagnostic tests, treatments, diagnostic impressions, planned evaluations.
   2. Educational/Vocational Function: Educational assessment and achievement versus potential, special needs, motivation, participation, goal orientation, eligibility for and availability of appropriate programs such as special education, vocational training.
   3. Cognitive Function: Developmental aspects (e.g., abstracting ability, egocentrism), level of organization, reality testing (including accuracy of perceptions, distinction between inner and outer stimuli, awareness of inner state and psychological mindedness), self-image, judgment, decision making, thought processes (including attention, concentration, memory, concept formation, language, anticipation, influence of primary versus secondary process on thinking, presence of looseness, tangentiality), abnormal thought content.
   4. Affective Function: Awareness of feelings, differentiation of feelings, ability to express feelings with range and appropriateness, intensity, predominant mood.
   5. Behavioral: Age appropriateness of behavior, responsibility for behavior, impulse control, ability to delay gratification, frustration tolerance, nature of impulse expression.
   6. Behavioral: Capacity for group function, capacity for cooperative play/work, object relations (including relationships with dependency figures, authority figures, peers, sexual object choice).
   7. Recreational Function: Small muscle and gross motor coordination, athletic ability and sense of fair play, special skills, use of unstructured time, community resources.
   8. Interests: Hobbies, sports, artistic endeavors.
   9. Strengths: Intellectual ability, scholastic or athletic competence, interpersonal skills, appearance.
  10. Family: Intactness, stability, involvement in treatment, motivation, communication, alliances, how dependency needs are met, separation, individua-

tion. A statement of goals, methods, and who is responsible should be included.

11. Legal Status: Guardian, court involvement.
12. Estimated Length of Stay: An attempt should be made to address this issue based on clinical status, family issues, and dispositional factors.
13. Prognosis: Should be addressed based on ongoing clinical assessment, constitutional factors, response to treatment, and external support systems.
14. Discharge Plan: Every attempt should be made to formulate a specific discharge plan at the earliest possible date, even prior to admission (including who will be involved, medications, and post-discharge treatment recommendations). Development of the plan should involve the resident and significant others.
15. Aftercare and Follow-up Plans: The transitional period following termination may require variable degrees of support for the individual patient (possibly including a structured plan for visits and telephone contacts), with particular attention paid to minimizing regression and facilitating development of new treatment alliances and relationships. Statement of specific goals, methods, and staff responsible should be made. Follow-up evaluation should be accomplished at some specified time (e.g., 6 months) by a designated staff person.

## RECOMMENDATIONS

1. Licensed mental health professionals should be intricately involved in the treatment of each resident.
2. Psychiatrists should be involved as consultants in three ways: patient-centered, staff-centered, and program-centered. They may be the individual therapists.
3. Attention should be directed to the transitional periods immediately prior to and following the actual admission to the facility to improve success of treatment and reduce recidivism.
4. Psychiatrist reviewers should be requested to make on-site visits to familiarize themselves with the residential treatment facilities.

5. Utilization review should be carried out with the goal of providing the patient with maximum therapeutic benefit, thus maximizing postdischarge adjustment and preventing unnecessary recidivism.
6. Health financing should encourage development of a full spectrum of treatment resources, thus providing the most appropriate treatment and making the most efficient use of the mental health dollar. To accomplish this goal, third-party payers should work with local and state funding sources.

## SUMMARY

The purpose of this chapter was to define residential treatment in its current form. After drawing a brief historical perspective, we attempted to show that residential treatment exists within a broad continuum of interrelated treatment services.

Without residential treatment existing as it does between acute hospital care and outpatient treatment, two very negative consequences would occur: 1) lengths of stay in hospitals would increase drastically, and 2) a very needy patient group would be deprived of the most appropriate treatment.

Since residential treatment is about one-third the cost of hospital treatment, it behooves everyone to give this level of care serious recognition.

Aftercare and follow-up statistics are beginning to show the efficacy and success of this form of treatment clearly. As more and more data are gathered, the case for residential treatment can only be strengthened.

# 10

# Confidentiality

*Daniel B. Borenstein, M.D.*

# Confidentiality

> *Whatsoever I shall see or hear concerning the life of men, in my attendance on the sick or even apart therefrom, which ought not to be noised abroad, I will keep silence thereon, counting such things to be as holy secrets.*
> —The Hippocratic Oath

C onfidentiality is essential for successful psychiatric treatment. Without it, patients would be hesitant to enter into a meaningful psychotherapeutic relationship. Yet, on close examination, it is evident that the private communications of patients to physicians are not completely protected from disclosure. This poses a special problem and concern for psychiatrists and their patients because of the stigma attached to psychiatric illness. As third parties provide additional financial coverage for these disorders, there is a concomitant requirement for increased professional accountability. The resulting right of fiscally responsible third parties to limited therapeutic information

175

conflicts with the patient's right to privacy and the physician's oath to keep communications "as holy secrets." Psychiatric peer review provides a means for the optimal resolution of these conflicting rights and requirements.

## DEFINITIONS

A definition of the concepts to be discussed in more detail may be helpful. *Privacy* refers to an individual's constitutional right to freedom from unauthorized intrusion by others. This right may be extended to include communications that are given in trust to another individual. The obligation to maintain the privacy of these communications is what is meant by *confidentiality*. Physician–patient confidentiality is an ethical requirement that the Greeks originated and formalized in their Hippocratic oath. It has been repeatedly reaffirmed in physicians' codes of ethics and is a requirement of most medical licensing statutes. It is important to note that private information revealed in this manner remains the property of the patient. When appropriate statutes are enacted, the confidential information is legally protected from disclosure. Such information is said to be *privileged* and is referred to as privileged communication, physician–patient privilege, and psychotherapist–patient privilege.

Since the individual retains the proprietory right to privileged communications, it follows that the patient alone has the right to disclose this information. The individual may do so, or may authorize other holders of the information to reveal it. Therefore, the sequence may be traced from privacy to confidentiality to privilege to voluntary relinquishment of privacy.

The final term to be considered here is *informed consent*. In general, for an individual to give informed consent to a procedure or action, the person must be provided with information about it, be aware of the potential consequences, and must consent freely. If the individual is unable to understand that to which he or she is consenting or if consent is obtained by deceit, fraud, or coercion, it cannot be considered informed consent.

# THERAPEUTIC CONSIDERATIONS

It is of interest that in Freud's writings he did not comprehensively address the issue of confidentiality. In fact, there
are no references to confidentiality in an index of Freud's
major publications (Strachey 1974). In contrast, subsequent psychiatrists have repeatedly stated their concern
about potential breaches of confidentiality and the need to
safeguard their patients' identities and communications.
Freedman (1980), in a well-known psychiatric textbook, observed that:

*All physicians are concerned with confidentiality, but the
sensibilities of psychiatrists are especially heightened in
regard to this issue. The patient, especially if involved in
any form of psychotherapy, must be assured beyond any
shadow of doubt that his or her communications to the
therapist will be held inviolate. Otherwise, treatment cannot proceed satisfactorily (p 3231).*

Freedman (1980) also emphasized that for therapy to
succeed, a patient must be confident that he or she can
disclose the "most intimate, embarrassing, humiliating experiences, thoughts, dreams, and fantasies" (p 3231). If the
patient is not convinced that these intimate revelations will
remain within the consulting room, there will be a significant (and at times insurmountable) resistance to therapy.
The need for confidentiality goes beyond the harmful effect
that disclosure could impose on the patient; it also invades
the private lives of individuals with whom the patient has
associated. The Group for the Advancement of Psychiatry
(1960) states that "among physicians, the psychiatrist has
a special need to maintain confidentiality. His capacity to
help his patients is completely dependent upon their willingness and ability to talk freely. . . . There is wide agreement that confidentiality is a sine qua non for successful
psychiatric treatment" (p 92). The report emphasizes that
confidentiality is central to psychiatric treatment. Shwed et
al (1979) concur, stating that "nowhere is confidentiality
more basic to a discipline than in psychiatry and psychotherapy. . . . Guarantees of confidentiality [are essential to
establish a therapeutic alliance between patient and psychi-

atrist for they allow the patient to] share increasingly intimate and difficult material with the therapist" (pp
447–448). Not only are these guarantees necessary, but,
"for the overly-sensitive or frankly paranoid patient any hint
that confidentiality has been violated will destroy the
therapeutic endeavor" (p 448).

There are other therapeutic reasons for maintaining
confidentiality. For example, confidentiality is necessary to
discourage secondary gain; it ensures that the psychiatrist
will not unknowingly participate in manipulating others in
the patient's extratherapeutic life (Dubey 1974). The need to
disclose insurance claims data may serve as a source of
resistance to progress within therapy. Patients may be hesitant to improve because they might experience this as a
threat to receiving third-party payments and thus inhibit
their ability to continue their treatment. They may experience an unconscious motivation to provide their psychiatrist with evidence of their sickness to justify their continued treatment. This establishes a paradox: the patient
remains mentally ill in order to try to get well. A recent
survey of psychiatric patients and nonpatients revealed a
significant concern that a psychiatrist might divulge confidential information concerning them. About one-third of
the nonpatients indicated that the possibility of a psychiatrist divulging confidential information would prevent them
from seeking psychotherapy (Lindenthal and Thomas
1982).

Psychiatry's special concern about confidentiality is reflected in Section 4 of the American Psychiatric Association's (APA) *Principles of Medical Ethics with Annotations
Especially Applicable to Psychiatry* (American Psychiatric
Association 1981), which are based on the AMA's code of
ethics. This section states that "a physician shall respect
the rights of patients, of colleagues, and of other health
professionals, and shall safeguard patient confidences
within the constraints of the law" (p 5). As noted above,
confidentiality is a matter of ethics rather than a legal requirement. Added weight is given to this principle of medical ethics through its 13 annotations. None of the other
sections receives this degree of attention and specificity.

A portion of the extreme concern that the psychiatric
community has in relation to psychotherapist–patient con-

fidentiality is related to the continuing stigma in our society attached to psychiatric illness and to a patient known to have seen a psychiatrist. It is reminiscent of the attitudes that have been expressed about patients who have leprosy or sexually transmitted disease. However, the deprecation of psychiatry is much more extensive; it encompasses the entire range of mental illness and contains within it the conviction that the individual is weak or inadequate. Furthermore, this phenomenon is widely recognized outside the psychiatric profession. The Privacy Protection Study Commission (1977), focusing specifically on personal privacy in our society, was fully aware of this prevailing attitude:

> One's own physician . . . may heartily approve of taking a minor or temporary problem to a psychiatrist, but the potential consequence of disclosing the mere fact that one has had psychiatric treatment are too well-known to need description (p 10).
> Because of the social stigma attached to mental and nervous disorders in our society, even the fact of admission to a psychiatric hospital or disclosure of the name of the attending physician in general hospital can have untoward consequences for an individual (p 286).

A study of the attitudes of supervisors toward present and potential employees receiving psychiatric help supports the Commission's conclusions: 55 percent of the supervisors indicated that they would have a negative attitude toward an employee who had seen a psychiatrist. Even if the employee had a good supervisory rating, the fact that the employee had received psychiatric care might hinder or rule out promotion for that individual (Melchiode and Jacobson 1976). One need only recall how the public revelation of Senator Thomas Eagleton's history of psychiatric care ended his candidacy for vice president of the United States in 1972. His case, among others, provides the rationale for public figures assuming pseudonyms when they enter psychiatric hospitals (Slovenko 1979).

Because of ethical and therapeutic concerns, psychoanalysts (in re Lifschuts 1970) and psychiatrists (Caesar v Mountanos 1976) have been willing to serve jail sentences for contempt of court rather than reveal the confidential information entrusted to them by their patients. This has been the case even though the psychotherapists received the patient's permission to disclose this information and were legally bound to do so. Another way in which this protectiveness has appeared is that the therapist reports less severe or less stigmatizing diagnoses on claims forms. Chodoff (1978) suggests that "when he or she is unwilling to make an accurate diagnosis because of considerations of confidentiality . . . a psychiatrist is likely to take refuge in writing bland diagnoses such as anxiety neurosis or depressive neurosis" (p 1142). These determinations, Chodoff maintains, will not threaten the therapeutic relationship. In addition, disclosure of the psychiatric care would be less damaging to the patient. This hypothesis was later confirmed in a study by Sharfstein et al. (1980). They compared the diagnoses from the Washington Psychiatric Society that were submitted on insurance claims forms with those that were submitted on confidential questionnaires. The claims forms contained the diagnosis of neurosis in 84.3 percent of the cases in comparison to 28.4 percent in the confidential study. In contrast, the claims forms contained the diagnosis of psychosis in 10.6 percent and personality disorder in 9.5 percent of the cases compared to 24.7 percent and 20.8 percent, respectively, in the confidential study. The authors' conclusion was that the less severe diagnoses were submitted to insurance companies because of fears about confidentiality and the stigma attached to diagnoses like schizophrenia and alcoholism.

There seems to be little doubt that diagnostic information submitted on claims forms is unreliable for peer review. However, as Chodoff (1978) observes, "the delicate fabric of the psychotherapeutic relationship, which depends on the honesty and integrity of the therapist, may be damaged in the atmosphere of collusion between the participants in making such diagnoses only to secure reimbursement" (pp 1142–1143). Useless diagnostic information on claims forms may be one of the reasons why third-party payers are increasingly demanding additional information. It is clear that there are a number of potentially destructive consequences to this well-meaning practice. The solution to this dilemma lies in the establishment of professional psychiatric peer review in which the identity of the patient is not revealed to the reviewers and the sensitive, therapeutic information is not disclosed to the third-party payers. Such an ideal system of peer review is described below.

The confidentiality of communications from psychiatric patients is threatened from many directions. Third-party payers, peer review structures, legal actions, and government agencies are eroding the exclusively dyadic psychiatrist—patient relationship. These intrusions have been disruptive and, occasionally, have led to an interruption or termination of a patient's treatment. The introduction of a new mental health insurance form, requesting more detailed information, led to patients refusing to start treatment, disruptions, and interruptions of ongoing treatment. The treating psychiatrists were so disturbed by the new form that they threatened legal action which led to the withdrawal of the form (Chodoff 1978).

Shwed et al. (1979) described how a routine Medicaid audit damaged patients' trust, feelings of confidentiality, and doctors' reputations; there were transference reactions and exacerbated emotional states. Uhill (1798) related how the deviations from confidentiality in the inpatient treatment of a patient with borderline personality led to acting out and premature termination of the treatment. Appendix H of the *APA's Confidentiality and Third Parties* (American Psychiatric Association 1975) lists 29 samples of reports from psychiatrists of injuries to patients as a result of breaches of confidentiality.

## BREACHES OF CONFIDENTIALITY

The doctor—patient relationship is invaded from many directions and at many levels. At times, confidential information is released voluntarily within ethical and legal boundaries, but it may also be obtained outside of physicians' and patients' control. Federal and state statutes require physicians to report births, deaths, communicable diseases, environmentally caused cancers, drug addiction, violence-related injuries, and child abuse. The justification for each of these intrusions in the medical care relationship is that society's need for information outweighs the individual's claim to personal privacy. Other intrusions include the required provision of information to third-party payers.

At a different level, information is revealed to professional peer review groups, professional review organizations (PROs), supervisors, and employers. Hospital records are audited and inspected by quality-control, cost-conscious, and regulatory groups. The billing, bookkeeping, and collection practices of physicians necessitate the disclosure of their patients' identities. Access to physicians' records may be obtained in criminal investigations and in legal actions. In addition, physicians may be required to testify in various court proceedings.

Psychiatrists are often employed to evaluate individuals and to report the findings of these evaluations. They may be called in as experts in insanity determinations, disability examinations, employment examinations, security clearance examinations, determinations of legal competence, and evaluation of suitability for various jobs. In all of these circumstances, prior to beginning the evaluation, the examining psychiatrist has a duty to inform the individual of the examination's purpose and lack of confidentiality. At times, to protect a patient or the community from imminent danger, the psychiatrist may determine it necessary to reveal confidential information. As a result of the Tarasoff case in California, psychiatrists must warn possible victims of a potentially dangerous patient (Tarasoff v Regents of the University of California 1976). This is a most unfortunate law because predicting dangerous behavior is unreliable and the patient's knowledge of this requirement will undoubtedly hinder the therapeutic process.

Concern about potential breaches of confidentiality has been heightened because of the extensive amount of personal information being stored. This is partially explained by the increasing use of computer data banks without adequate safeguards. At the same time, more sensitive information is at risk within the records of psychiatric hospitals and clinics because significantly more data is collected in order to pass accreditation and quality assurance reviews, as well as to justify third-party payments.

During the 1970s, in addition to the legal and required breaches of confidentiality, the public learned of criminal intrusions into private records. The most glaring example was the burglary of Dr. Fielding's office in search of Dr. Ellsberg's psychiatric records. This felony was revealed during the Watergate investigation.

Plaut (1974) suggested that the degree of required intrusion into the psychiatrist–patient relationship is directly related to the amount of civil authority vested in the psychiatrist. Where this authority is extensive, as in performing commitment procedures, in criminal and civil law suits, and in psychiatric hospitalizations, it is reasonable to expect many exceptions to the physician–patient privilege. He placed psychoanalysis at the other end of the spectrum in which there would be no third-party payer, no civil authority vested in the psychoanalyst, and maximal protection of the patient's communications, similar to that of a priest–penitent. Between the two extremes, Plaut visualized the psychotherapeutic relationship with limited civil authority and limited breaches of confidentiality.

## PRIVACY RIGHTS

The United States Constitution did not explicitly guarantee the right to privacy. It has been one of the most ill-defined concepts in American jurisprudence, developing through a patchwork of common and statutory law. A late nineteenth-century definition of privacy explained that it is the right "to be let alone" (Cooley 1888, p 280). In 1928, Justice Brandeis used this definition in a U.S. Supreme Court case dealing with personal privacy (Olmstead v United States 1928). His dissenting opinion stated that "the makers of our Constitution . . . sought to protect Americans in their beliefs, their thoughts, their emotions and their sensations. They conferred . . . the right to be let alone—the most comprehensive of rights and the right most valued by civilized men" (p 478). Thirty-seven years later, the U.S. Supreme Court affirmed the existence of a constitutional right to privacy (Griswold v Connecticut 1965). The first physician–patient privilege statute was enacted in New York in 1928 (Guttmacher 1960). Since that time, according to Slovenko (1979), 36 states have enacted similar statutes. Georgia, the first state to recognize the importance of privileged communications in psychiatric treatment, passed a statute in 1959, which granted privileged communication to patients in psychiatric treatment (Group for the Advancement of Psychiatry 1960). Only a few states have passed specific legislation protecting the psychotherapist–patient privilege. These include California, Connecticut, Florida, Georgia, Illinois, Kentucky, and Massachusetts. Unfortunately, the physician–patient privilege and psychotherapist–patient privilege are riddled with many exceptions and qualifications. "The psychotherapist–patient privilege, like the medical privilege before it, offers a shield that looks more like a sieve . . . virtually nothing about a patient in litigation is shielded by the shield (Slovenko 1979, p 452). In strictly federal cases, there is no psychotherapist–patient privilege.

## INFORMED CONSENT

Medical information consent is usually discussed in terms of consent of treatment. In the present context, it may be considered as consent for both somatic and psychological forms of psychiatric treatment. It must also be considered in relation to a patient's waiving the psychiatrist–patient privilege for the release of confidential information or in consenting to the release of psychiatric records. Meisel et al. (1977) placed the legal antecedents to modern informed consent as far back as the late eighteenth century. However, its development into a full-blown doctrine did not occur until the early 1960s.

Informed consent must be given voluntarily, that is, without inducements, coercion, fraud, or deceit. The patient must be provided with information and must be competent to understand it (Joling 1974; Meisel et al. 1977). The information must be provided in simple language and it should explain the risks, benefits, alternatives, and likely results of a decision not to consent. "Patients are presumed to have the capacity to comprehend the information with which they are provided to the extent that a 'reasonable' person would understand it" (Meisel et al. 1977, p 287). The patient must not be hampered by any condition, including psychiatric illness, that would interfere with understanding equivalent to that of an average person. The law regarding informed consent is changing and evolving and is "particularly complicated, both because of the right-to-refuse-treatment litigation and because our patients may lack the capacity to give informed consent as a result of their mental illness" (Stone 1979, p 323). There remains the theoretical question as to whether or not an individual can ever be fully enough informed to provide this degree of consent. Furthermore, most empirical evidence demonstrates that even when patients are given complete and appropriate information, most do not comprehend it or retain it (Stone 1979).

## MEDICAL RECORDS

The APA has had an understandable and an abiding interest in the confidentiality of medical records. This is evident in its position statement (American Psychiatric Association 1972); its task force report (American Psychiatric Association 1975); its leadership in the formation of the National Commission on Confidentiality of Health Records, which was incorporated in 1976 (Spingarn 1975); and its model law (American Psychiatric Association 1979). We have previously alluded to the numerous opportunities for breaches of confidentiality regarding the hospital records of psychiatric patients. This section will focus on the appropriate requirements for authorized release of medical records, including psychiatric records, and the suggested requirements to provide patients with access to psychiatric records. The APA Task Force on *Confidentiality and Third Parties* correctly states that blanket consent for release of unspecified information is not acceptable (American Psychiatric Association 1975). It encourages the requirement of separate informed consent for each disclosure. The problem, as discussed in the previous section, is that in many situations, psychiatric patients cannot meet the requirements for genuine informed consent. In addition, patients are usually unaware of the specific contents of medical and psychiatric records. Therefore, they may consent to the release of this information without completely understanding it or without the ability to evaluate the full potential impact of its release. Providing patients access to their medical records will help rectify this situation.

The "Model Law on Confidentiality of Health and Social Service Records" (American Psychiatric Association 1979) recommends requirements for authorized disclosures. It also identifies those disclosures that: are permissable without authorization, including those within a service-providing facility; involve a supervisory relationship; are for pro-

tection of another from serious injury or disease; pertain to
billing and claims procedures; are legally required through
court action, such as the patient–litigant exception; and
involve court-ordered examinations.

The Privacy Protection Study Commission (1977) also
recommends a valid authorization to permit the disclosure
or release of medical records. Both the APA model law and
the Privacy Commission's recommendations require that
the authorization (1) be in writing, (2) be signed by the
patient or an authorized representative, (3) specify the
nature and content of the information to be disclosed, (4)
specify to whom the information is to be disclosed, and (5)
specify the specific purpose for which the information may
be used. The APA model law allows for the patient or an
authorized representative to withdraw such consent at any
time in writing. The Privacy Commission added a requirement to include the medical care provider among those
being designated to disclose this information. It also requires that specifications be provided describing the use(s)
of the information not only at the time of disclosure but its
future application(s) as well. Furthermore, it suggests the
inclusion of an expiration date, generally not exceeding one
year.

Through the combined efforts of dedicated professional
and community leaders, plus vigorous individual lobbying
in Illinois, a new state statute, the Mental Health and Developmental Disabilities Confidentiality Act, was enacted in
1979 (Foster 1980). This comprehensive act incorporates
the above-noted provisions and may be considered a model
for similar legislation in other states.

The Privacy Act of 1974 (5 USC) led the way toward
patient access to all records, including medical records
within federal programs. The Privacy Act also established
the Privacy Protection Study Commission, which recommends "that upon request, an individual who was a subject
of a medical record maintained by a medical-care provider,
or another responsible person designated by the individual,
be allowed to have access to that medical records, including
an opportunity to see and copy it" (Privacy Protection Study
Commission 1977, p 298). The Department of Health, Education, and Welfare, the Department of Defense, and the
Veterans' Administration have all provided for indirect access to records.

Patient access provisions in the APA model law follow the Privacy Commission's recommendations to allow the individual to contest the accuracy of the record or correct inaccurate information by adding a statement setting forth what the individual believes to be an accurate or a more complete record where there appears to be a deficiency. The model law also permits the patient to appoint another clinician of his or her choice who would have access to the record when the treating physician is concerned that disclosure of the recorded information would be detrimental to the patient. In January 1983, a California statute went into effect which permits a patient access to his or her medical records, including indirect access when the physician is concerned about the information being harmful to the patient (Health and Safety Code 1983). Illinois and Massachusetts are among the states that have enacted parallel statutes. It is probable that many states will pass similar legislation in the near future.

The concept of "personal notes" has existed in the legal profession for some time. These notes may contain information from confidential sources; information that may be harmful to the client; sensitive information the client has disclosed to the attorney; and the attorney's speculations. The advantage of these notes is that they are considered to be the work product and personal property of the attorney and, as such, are not subject to discovery in judicial, administrative, or legislative proceedings. A similar concept for psychiatrists is included in the APA model law. It may be important and advantageous to establish this method of note taking alongside more formal records in view of potentially required disclosure of and patient access to the primary records.

## INSURANCE RECORDS

The most frequent breach of patient–psychiatrist confidentiality occurs through the release of insurance records. They are, therefore, seen as the largest source of risk and harm to psychiatric patients. Prior to 1960, psychiatric insurance coverage was restricted to inpatient benefits and was quite limited (Fowler 1978). By 1980, between 85 and 90 percent of the population had some form of health cover-

age. The more extensive inpatient and outpatient coverages
come under intense scrutiny by the insurance industry and
employers because they represent increased financial risk
to these groups. Insurers and their support organizations
are one of the largest, if not the largest, collectors of personally identifiable information in the United States. Despite
these developments, relatively little attention has been
focused on the issues of confidentiality in the management
of industry records (Skipper 1979). The industry as a whole
has made no provisions for special handling of psychiatric
records. However, these sensitive records have received
more careful consideration in some individual insurance
companies and insurance programs.

Another concern is the use of blanket consent forms for
release of confidential information, a standard policy within
the industry. These forms are signed when individuals apply for insurance coverage. They are regularly used by inves-
tigative agencies within the insurance industry to look into
individuals' past and present medical history and treatment, including psychiatric treatment. The same forms are
used to request release of information for treatment that
occurs after the insurance coverage goes into effect. Use of
this authorization does not limit further dissemination of
the disclosed information.

Disclosure of personal information often occurs when
employee insurance plans are administered through personnel departments where supervisors and the idly curious
may have access to them. A more appropriate arrangement
routes health insurance claims directly to insurance companies. Some carriers have supplied monthly reports containing identifying information to employers. In other instances, employers have obtained insurance records on
request.

It is less well-known that personally identifiable information is often passed around within the insurance industry. Prior to the mid-1970s, few people were aware of the
existence of the Medical Information Bureau (MIB), which
collects and stores medical information on individuals and
shares this information freely within the insurance industry. In 1975, in response to criticism for its secretive ways,
the MIB instituted a requirement that insurance applicants
be informed about the bureau. Similarly, a number of insurers have voluntarily adopted a policy restricting the sharing

of personally identifiable information with other insurers. However, there are essentially no legal restrictions to the free flow of information within the insurance industry. Only one federal law, the 1970 Fair Credit Reporting Act (15 USC), affects the record-keeping practices of the insurance industry. This law has little effect on the handling of medical records.

The Privacy Protection Study Commission (1977) makes similar recommendations for the authorization to release insurance records, as previously noted in regard to medical records. Such authorization must be given freely, should be in plain language, and be dated. It should also specify the individuals and institutions authorized to disclose information, the nature of the information begin authorized for disclosure, the individuals or institutions to whom the information may be disclosed, and the purpose the information may be used for. In addition, it should include a specific expiration date no later than one year after the authorization or two years after the issuance of the policy. The Privacy Commission maintained that "the enforceable expectation of confidentiality it recommends must be implemented by federal statute" (p 185). The Privacy Commission did not address the free flow of information within the insurance industry in a more direct manner.

The National Association of Insurance Commissioners (NAIC) has proposed a NAIC Insurance Information and Privacy Protection Model Act (National Association of Insurance Commissioners 1980). The proposed model contained serious inadequacies. It continues to permit the unhindered flow of information within the insurance industry and it includes permission for 16 forms of "reasonably necessary" disclosure to individuals or organizations outside of an insurance company without written authorization. One of these permissable disclosures would be to a professional peer review organization. It also proposes that authorizations signed for the purpose of collecting information for health insurance claims remain valid for the entire term of the policy. In regard to access to recorded personal information, the proposal places insurance institutions or agents in the position of deciding whether records should be released directly to the individual or to a medical professional designated by that individual. This decision should be made by the treating physician. The NAIC model is a significant step in the right direction, but does not contain the safeguards for the confidential handling of individual information that both professionals and patients desire. Despite these limitations, the model act has become law in eight states: Arizona, California, Connecticut, Illinois, Kansas, Montana, Nevada, and Virginia. It does not provide for any special handling or storage of psychiatric records.

In contrast, the District of Columbia's Mental Health Information Act (1978) was enacted "to establish safeguards to maintain the confidentiality of mental health information. . . . " Conforming with the recommendations of both the APA model act and the Privacy Protection Study Commission, it also addresses and spells out appropriate mechanisms of limited disclosure for fee collection, research, auditing, and program evaluation. It contains unique features such as establishing the right to anonymity for patients and others in court records that contain mental health information. The act also includes the important provision for both civil liberties and criminal penalties for violations. Furthermore, it deals with the thorny problem of mental health records released to police departments. This section requires that such records be maintained separately; they do not become a part of any permanent policy record. They must be destroyed if no judicial action is pending, or at the expiration of the statute of limitations.

A most significant section of the District of Columbia Act outlines the procedure for limited disclosure to third-party payers. This section permits authorized disclosure of administrative information, diagnostic information, the voluntary or involuntary status of the patient, the reason for admission or continuing treatment, and prognosis for the estimated duration of the treatment. If the third-party payer has additional questions about the appropriateness of aspects of the patient's care, it may, with additional valid authorization, request an independent review of the patient's mental health information by nontreating mental health professionals. However, mental health information disclosed for the purpose of review may not be disclosed to the third-party payer.

Some insurance companies have recognized the need for special handling of psychiatric records and send them directly to the company's medical director or a designee in the central office. These records are seen by a limited number of specially trained personnel and are stored separately from other medical records. The Aetna Insurance Company and its former medical director, Dr. William Guillette, were early, active participants in the development of these special procedures. A group of insurance companies that are members of the Health Insurance Association of America (HIAA) participated in the development of an APA coding project that would have permitted psychiatrists to submit claims information in the form of a code symbol without providing specific and detailed information about each patient. The code provides a prediction of both the severity of the illness and the anticipated duration of treatment, but it does not include a specific diagnosis. Although this was acceptable to the HIAA, and was shown to be effective in a field trial, it is not widely accepted by the insurance industry.

## APA PEER REVIEW ACTIVITIES

In the early 1970s, several APA district branch peer review committees developed sophisticated and confidential peer review mechanisms and procedures. The system created by the Southern California Psychiatric Society (1977) provided both confidential peer review and voluntary binding arbitration through an agreement with a national insurance company. The procedures were developed in the spirit of cooperation to assist the company in resolving disputed insurance claims and to assist the therapist and the patient by minimizing the intrusion into the treatment process. At the same time, they ensured that reviews would be done by peers who were skilled in and knowledgeable about the treatment being evaluated. A set of principles of psychiatric peer review were derived from these experiences and became the foundation for subsequent APA peer review activities.

In July 1977, the APA contracted with the Civilian Health and Medical Plan of the Uniformed Services (CHAMPUS) to provide peer review services. The objections and concerns about the intrusions of peer review and the potential breaches of confidentiality that were anticipated delayed implementation of the government contract until August 1979. In the same year, a number of articles ex-

pressing these concerns appeared on the front page of
*Psychiatric News* (Herrington 1979; McDonald 1979a,
1979b). In mid-1979, the first commercial contract was
signed with the Aetna Insurance Company; it became effective at the same time as CHAMPUS. The two initial projects
led to the fully developed APA Peer Review Program, which
began in 1980. It has continued to provide peer review for
the federal CHAMPUS program and a number of commercial carriers. As of December 1984, the APA had 26 contracts with insurance companies or brokers. The signed
memorandum of understanding between the carrier and
the APA established a number of mechanisms for confidential handling and storage of sensitive clinical information.
Previous efforts to initiate these changes within the insurance industry met with limited success. The agreements
with the APA provide a method for instituting these important changes.

A detailed presentation of the APA peer review procedure will not be described. However, the issues involving
confidentiality are discussed in this section. When a claim
is questioned, the medical director obtains additional
clinical information on a mental health treatment report
(MHTR). These reports are solicited from the treating physician and sent directly to the medical director. The clinical
information is not circulated through claim clerks, to the
patient's employer, or to any other agency within or without
the insurance company. In addition, these forms are not
processed through the employee's personnel department
and do not become a part of other medical claims records.
Treatment reports are destroyed when they are no longer
required to process a claim. Furthermore, the "Memorandum of Understanding" prohibits any portion of a report
from being stored in electronic data banks. None of the
information obtained during a review is released without
appropriate legal authority. The identity of both the patient
and the treating physician is removed from all treatment
reports and supplemental material prior to its being forwarded to the APA for peer review. The APA Peer Review
Office assigns each case to three peer reviewers for commercial reviews. The reviewers' identities are not disclosed to
the carrier. Despite these security measures, some psychiatrists continue to be concerned about potential leaks of
sensitive clinical information from the MHTRs, which are

stored in both the APA Peer Review Office and the carrier's files for extended periods of time. The carrier's files, of course, contain personally identifiable information.

The most frequently used MHTR requests the following information:

1. The patient's initial reason for seeking treatment and previous psychiatric history and treatment.
2. The patient's current condition, including duration and severity of functional impairment and stress factors.
3. Results of a mental status examination.
4. When applicable, date and significant findings of physical and psychological examinations, including pertinent laboratory tests.
5. (For the diagnosis of alcoholism) the results of neurological, liver function, and chemical screens.
6. Current treatment goals.
7. Modality of treatment, including frequency, length of sessions, and anticipated duration.
8. Medications, including dosage and date.
9. Collaterial contacts and adjunctive therapies.
10. Rationale for psychotherapy sessions occurring more than two times per week.

Although not required, there is a mechanism in the APA procedures for informing the patient of the extent of information being provided to the carrier and the purpose for which it is to be used. Informed consent and patient access are left to the discretion of the provider. The clinical data on the MHTR may be shown to the patient if the therapist wishes to share it. To facilitate this process, each request for an MHTR is accompanied by a limited release form that may be used by the therapist to obtain the patient's authorization to release pertinent information. The form states the following:

> *I understand that this information will be used solely to review the necessity and quality of care received by the patient, and that this review process will include a panel of psychiatrists or psychologists acting for their professional associations. I further understand that the patient's identity will not be disclosed to this panel nor will the information released under this authorization be used or disclosed*

*for any other purpose in individually identifiable form
without written consent, unless expressly permitted or required by law.*

*I know this authorization may be revoked at any time by
written notice to [insurance company], but this will not
affect any action taken or information already released.
Otherwise, this authorization will be valid until final payment of the claim for benefits to which it relates.*

*I also know that I have the right to ask for and receive a
copy of this authorization. I agree that a photographic copy
of this authorization will be as valid as the original.*

The limited release form was developed by the APA and
Aetna Life and Casualty Company in response to members'
complaints about being asked to release information based
on a general release statement signed by patients as a part
of the routine claims process. It was hoped that this form
would address concerns about informed consent and patient access.

The patient is not told how long information will remain in the carrier's files and is given no guarantee that it
will be destroyed. However, the agreements between the
insurance companies and the APA asks that the material be
destroyed "when no longer required in connection with the
processing of a claim."

Also, there is a probability that these records would be
subject to subpoena in legal proceedings and disclosed during criminal investigations. State insurance departments
and federal agencies can insist on access to insurance company records. Although there is the potential for leaks of
information, to date there have been no significant known
or reported breaches of confidentiality in the APA peer review program.

An analysis of the first year and a half of the APA–Aetna
peer review activities reveals that only one of ten cases
selected for submittal of a MHTR was referred for peer review (Rosner 1980). Therefore, sensitive and extensive
clinical information was collected 90 percent of the time to
determine that it was not actually needed for peer review. An
APA peer review survey of 2,690 psychiatrists yielding 1,092
responses reported that 58.1 percent had patients who de-
clined to file insurance claims, and 13.7 percent had pa-

tients who terminated their treatment because of the additional information requested on the MHTRs (American Psychiatric Association 1980).

## AN IDEAL PEER REVIEW PROGRAM

The ideal peer review program, as previously suggested, provides a system of professional psychiatric peer review in which the identity of the patient is not disclosed to reviewers and in which sensitive, detailed therapeutic information is not revealed to third-party payers. This program minimizes the intrusion into the psychotherapeutic relationship. At the same time, the third party is assured that the treatment is both appropriate and necessary, or informed that it is inappropriate and requires modification or discontinuation. The insurance company would be responsible for obtaining genuine informed consent for this procedure. Using its internal claims criteria, the insurance company would request peer review when it was concerned about a particular claim. At that point, the insurance company would assign a code number to the patient and request that the treating psychiatrist submit a confidential report to the chairperson of the local APA district branch peer review committee. This request instructs the psychiatrist to omit any information that would reveal the identity of the psychiatrist, the patient, or the treatment facility, if any. The clinical information should be identified by the assigned code number. The psychiatrist is asked to provide his or her name and address on a separate face sheet containing the assigned code number and the name and address of the medical director of the third-party carrier. This face sheet is removed by the peer review chair. The APA Peer Review Office facilitates a liaison with and assists carriers by identifying the appropriate local peer review committee chair. The chairperson would review the MHTR and assign it to three appropriately skilled and knowledgeable anonymous reviewers. Each district branch develops its own procedure for establishing qualified panels of reviewers, although the APA may be called on for assistance. The peer review chairperson may request additional information from the treating psychiatrist if it is needed for an accurate determination. The three reviewers would evaluate the clinical information independently. One of them could be appointed to collate and summarize their findings. If the reviewers needed assistance in clarifying aspects of the appropriateness of care, they could present their dilemma to the entire peer review committee. The final summary, with the reviewers' opinions, is given to the chairperson who sends copies containing the assigned code number to both the third-party medical director and the treating psychiatrist. The original and all copies of the clinical material are returned to the treating psychiatrist. An alternate procedure would be to destroy all clinical material after a specified period of time, not to exceed a few months.

Since a number of insurance carriers have shown a flexibility and willingness to work with peer review committees and the initial experience with the APA program has been positive, it may be time to move toward a more ideal peer review system. It is likely that a number of patients have been denied, or have avoided, treatment because of their concerns about the potential breaches of confidentiality contained within the present APA peer review program. There is no doubt that treating psychiatrists tend to minimize the extent of a patient's psychiatric illness in reports that are submitted to insurance companies. Some claims have been denied because a watered-down diagnosis appeared to be of insufficient severity to warrant coverage. Psychiatrists would feel more comfortable with and willing to provide clinical information to anonymous respected colleagues for a limited period of time. It seems reasonable to attempt to alter at least a portion of the APA peer review agreements, incorporating the more confidential, less risky procedure. The "ideal" approach has been used effectively by some of the district branches in the past.

## LEGAL INTRUSIONS

A number of intrusions into confidential records and the doctor–patient relationship have been outlined in the previous sections of this chapter. Most have been permitted by law or required by regulations. In addition, one needs to consider the legal actions that pose a direct threat to professional peer review records. The legal issues are discussed in more detail in another chapter. At least 40 states have enacted statutes that grant confidentiality to peer review records, and limit their discoverability and admissibility in varying degrees (Dunn and Holbrook 1981). The general rationale behind these laws is to promote open discussion by peer review members without their feeling threatened. This protection would obviously enhance the effectiveness of any peer review procedure. Even in the absence of such protective state statutes, the courts have stated that there is a public interest in maintaining confidentiality of these records in order to improve the quality of patient care (Kucera 1981).

One must be aware of the advocates for increased accountability who demand the release of psychiatric records to prevent fraud and abuse (Slovenko 1979). Other critics have suggested that statutes that protect the confidentiality of peer review records are unconstitutional and unwise (Dunn 1978). In the ever-changing legal climate, laws vary from state to state and are subject to evolution and revision. The variations in societal attitudes toward privacy and accountability mandate careful monitoring of both statutory and common law in each state in order to be fully aware of increased protection of, or invasion into, psychiatric peer review proceedings.

## SUMMARY

An overview of the special concerns of psychiatrists in regard to confidentiality has been presented with particular emphasis on third-party intrusions into the doctor—patient relationship. Professional psychiatric peer review is viewed as a method for improving the quality of care and answering the demands for professional accountability. At the same time, it assists third-party payers to meet their fiscal responsibilities in funding psychiatric treatment that is medically necessary and appropriately delivered with minimal intrusion into the therapeutic relationship. Peer review for troublesome cases substantially reduces the third party's risk in claims disputes and potential litigation.

The APA peer review program is described with both its strengths and its weaknesses. A more ideal peer review program is presented in some detail. In the opinion of the author, the proposed program would minimize the risks for breaches of confidentiality, would keep the psychiatric profession in control of sensitive information, and would provide as high a quality of peer review as presently exists in the APA program, if not higher. Psychiatrists and third-party payers are encouraged to work together to improve the peer review process and procedures.

# REFERENCES

American Psychiatric Association: Position statement on the need for preserving confidentiality of medical records in any national health care system. Am J Psychiatry 128:1349, 1972

American Psychiatric Association: Confidentiality and Third Parties: Task Force Report. Washington, DC, American Psychiatric Association, 1975

American Psychiatric Association: Model law on confidentiality of health and social service records. Am J Psychiatry 136:138–144, 1979

American Psychiatric Association: APA Peer Review Survey: Preliminary Findings. Washington, DC, American Psychiatric Association, 1980

American Psychiatric Association: Principles of Medical Ethics with Annotations Especially Applicable to Psychiatry. Washington, DC, American Psychiatric Association, 1981

Caesar v Mountanos, 542 F. 2d 1064 (9th Cir 1976)

Chodoff P: Psychiatry and the fiscal third party. Am J Psychiatry 135:10, 1141–1147, 1978

Cooley T: A Treatise on the Law of Torts or the Wrongs which Arise Independent of Contract, 2nd Ed. Chicago, Callaghan and Company, 1888

Dubey J: Confidentiality as a requirement of the therapist: technical necessities for absolute privilege in psychotherapy. Am J Psychiatry 131:1093–1096, 1974

Dunn L: Peer review: a secret affair? Trustee 31:9–11, 13, 1978

Dunn L, Holbrook R: Legal issues concerning peer review documents. Topics in Health Record Management 2:9–16, 1981

Fair Credit Reporting Act of 1970, Sec 1981, 15 USC 1681a–1681t, (1970)

Foster L: State confidentiality laws: the Illinois act as a model for new legislation in other states. Am J Orthopsychiatry 50:659–665, 1980

Fowler D: The psychiatrist and health insurance claims review. Am J Psychiatry 39:519–522, 1978

Freedman AM: Confidentiality, in Comprehensive Textbook of Psychiatry. Edited by Kaplan H, Freedman A, Sadock B. Baltimore, Williams & Wilkins Co, 1980

Griswold v Connecticut, 381 US 479 (1965)

Group for the Advancement of Psychiatry: Confidentiality and Privileged Communications in the Practice of Psychiatry (Rep. No. 45, 1960) New York, Group for the Advancement of Psychiatry, 1960

Guttmacher M: The Mind of the Murderer. New York, Farrar, Straus & Budahy, 1960

Health and Safety Code, CA, Secs 25250–25258 (1983)

Herrington B: Broad concern seen for records confidentiality. Psychiatric News 14:1,8,9, 1979

In re Lifschuts, No. 2 Cal 3d 415, 467 P 2d 557 (1970)

Joling R: Informed consent, confidentiality and privilege in psychiatry: legal implications. Bull Am Acad Psychiatry Law 11:107–110, 1974

Kucera W: Discovery and admissibility: the use of peer review reports before and during trial. Journal of the American Association of Nurse Anesthetists 49:437–438, 1981

Lindenthal J, Thomas C: Psychiatrists, the public and confidentiality. J Nerv Ment Dis 170:319–323, 1982

McDonald M: Dispute focuses on CHAMPUS privacy. Psychiatric News 14:1,4,5,7, 1979a

McDonald M: Peer review dispute unsettling. Psychiatric News 14:1,26,39, 1979b

Meisel A, Roth L, Lidz C, Toward a model of the legal doctrine of informed consent. Am J Psychiatry 134:285–289, 1977

Melchiode C, Jacobson M: Psychiatric treatment: a barrier to employment progress. J Occup Med 18:98–101, 1976

Mental Health Information Act, Chapter 20, Section 6-2001-2076, District of Columbia (1978)

National Association of Insurance Commissioners: NAIC Insurance Information and Privacy Protection Model Act. Kansas City, Missouri, National Association of Insurance Commissioners, 1980

Olmstead v United States, 277 US 438 (1928)

Plaut E: A perspective on confidentiality. Am J Psychiatry 131:1021–1024, 1974

The Privacy Act of 1974, Sec 5 USC Sec 552a

Privacy Protection Study Commission: Personal Privacy in an Information Society: Report of the Privacy Protection Study Commission. Washington, DC, U.S. Government Printing Office, 1977

Rosner B: Psychiatrists, confidentiality, & insurance claims. Hastings Cent Rep 10:5–7, 1980

Sharfstein S, Towery O, Milowe I: Accuracy of diagnostic information submitted to an insurance company. Am J Psychiatry 137:70–73, 1980

Shwed H, Kuvin S, Baliga R: Medical audit: crisis in confidentiality and the patient–psychiatrist relationship. Am J Psychiatry 136:447–450, 1979

Skipper H: The privacy implications of insurers' information practices. Journal of Risk and Insurance 46:9–32, 1979

Slovenko R: Accountability and abuse of confidentiality in the practice of psychiatry. Int J Law Psychiatry 2:431–454, 1979

Southern California Psychiatric Society: Principles of Psychiatric Peer Review. Los Angeles, Southern California Psychiatric Society, 1977

Spingarn N: Confidentiality: A Report of the 1974 Conference on Confidentiality of Health Records. Washington, DC, American Psychiatric Association, 1975

Stone A: Informed consent: special problems for psychiatry. Hosp Community Psychiatry 30:321–328, 1979

Strachey J ed: The Standard Edition of the Complete Psychological Works of Sigmund Freud. London, Hogarth Press, 1974

Tarasoff v Regents of the University of California et al, 17 Cal 3d 425, 551 P 2d 334 (1976)

Uhill A: Deviations from confidentiality and the therapeutic holding environment. Int J Psychoanal Psychother 7:208–219, 1978

# 11

# Some Results of Peer Review

*Gary L. Shepherd, M.D.*

# Some Results of Peer Review

Psychiatric peer review activities began in the early 1970s. The increase in health care benefits and complexity of the health care system created a need for these activities. Organized psychiatry responded to these needs through activity at the local district branch level, the state level, and the national association level.

For many third-party payers, the effectiveness of therapeutic approaches in psychiatry seemed difficult to assess. The understanding of psychological concepts and their application to the treatment of an individual have always been difficult for those not trained in the discipline. Psychiatric diagnoses and variations in lengths of stay for given diagnoses in different geographical areas are debatable issues within psychiatry. In addition, they may be sources of confusion for third-party payers.

Through its component structure, the American Psychiatric Association (APA) devised a system of psychiatric peer review resulting in the development, refinement, and application of criteria and standards as valid in one part of the country as in another. These criteria are not rule books but rather useful guidelines that do not interfere with individualized treatment program for patients receiving care. These criteria are contained in the *Manual of Psychiatric Peer Review* (American Psychiatric Association 1981). The manual addresses issues pertaining to medical necessity and appropriateness of care, as well as other significant issues in the field of clinical psychiatry. APA Peer Review Committee members and consultants periodically revise and update the manual.

In addition, there is a national panel of psychiatrist peer reviewers nominated from each district branch that provides professional oversight and monitoring of both inpatient and outpatient psychiatric care. The peer reviewers (themselves practicing psychiatrists) treat patients of all ages and represent the major treatment modalities. As a result, the development of diagnostic and treatment criteria and the existence of experienced peer reviewers has helped psychiatry to earn the respect of both public and private third-party payers. Peer review promotes accountability, thereby increasing the profession's credibility.

The profession is only beginning to address peer review's cost effectiveness statistically. However, when quality and medical necessity (as determined by the profession) are present in medical care, there is potential for cost reduction through efficacious resource utilization. Organized American psychiatry believes that a quality assurance system that includes peer review is the best way to accomplish this. The findings and statistics developed to this point indicate that this premise is correct.

## LOCAL LEVEL

Numerous peer review activities have developed at the district branch level. These activities have all had an impact on the national program and on third-party payers. This chapter discusses only one activity as an example of the results of peer review at the local level. The San Diego project is also the one with which I am most familiar. Briefly, the San Diego project was designed to review all hospital admissions in San Diego County hospitals (approximately 1,600) for Civilian Health and Medical Program of the Uniformed Services (CHAMPUS) patients with a DSM-III (American Psychiatric Association 1980) diagnosis. The project operated for the period 1 July 1977 to 1 January 1983 and was administered by the San Diego Psychiatric Society, a district branch of the APA.

An evaluation of this review project yields important information. During the 5½-year study, the number of available hospital beds remained essentially unchanged for the adult psychiatric population. Data from the Office of CHAMPUS (OCHAMPUS) indicate that during the project's tenure, its beneficiary population in San Diego County probably increased. Adult (18 and older) population statistics collected during the 5 years of the study clearly show a significant decrease in number of admissions each year until they begin to plateau in the fifth year (Shepherd and Hubbard 1983). The total decrease in admissions was 25.9%. The mean length of stay increased by 0.3 days. (The reason for this increase will be discussed later.) These statistics demonstrate a major decrease in total hospital stays. If this decrease in inpatient days is converted into dollars, a savings for adult inpatient psychiatric care of $6.5 to $8 million can be demonstrated over the 5½ years of the project. This is believed to be a conservative estimate.

Another important finding relates to an identified shift in the types of patients admitted during the project. The ratio of patients admitted with psychotic diagnoses versus those identified with neurotic diagnoses significantly increased (Shepherd and Hubbard 1983). This was a real shift. With the comprehensive nature of the review, it was not possible to "hide" patients' diagnoses. Thus the percentage of persons admitted with a diagnosis of psychosis or major affective disorder increased and the percentage of patients with a neurotic diagnosis decreased. Those who were admitted seemed to be more severely ill than previous patient populations.

This phenomenon was discussed at many hospital staff meetings and with many individual psychiatrists. The psychiatrists reported that this phenomenon probably occurred because the criteria for admission had become more stringent. Therefore, they began working with patients on an outpatient basis when previously they would have sought hospitalization. Providers discovered that they could indeed safely and adequately handle many of these patients on an outpatient basis and patients still received appropriate care. The use of partial hospitalization and other alternatives to hospitalization were also considered more frequently.

The data were examined to verify validity. The second quarter in 1977 was compared to the same quarter in 1981. The results supported staff observations. Overall numbers of admissions had decreased (Shepherd and Hubbard 1983). Three diagnostic classifications—schizophrenic disorder, major affective disorders, and dysthymic disorder (depressive neurosis)—were compared. The largest percentage admission decrease was in those patients with dysthymic disorder. There was an increase in the percentage of admissions for those with diagnoses of schizophrenic disorders and of major affective disorders. To determine whether patients indeed were more severely ill when hospitalized, the number of days in "intensive care," the number of "72-hour holds" obtained, and the number of "14-day certifications" obtained from one quarter in 1977 were compared to the same quarter in 1981. A significant increase would support staff observations.

**Table 1.**  Admission Statistics for 1977 and 1981

| Year | ICU Days | 72-Hour Holds | 14-Day Certifications |
|------|----------|---------------|-----------------------|
| 1977 | 302      | 13            | 3                     |
| 1981 | 443      | 34            | 10                    |

Between 1977 and 1981, there was a 46.7 percent increase in the number of ICU days, a 161.5 percent increase in 72-hour holds, and a 233.3 percent increase in 14-day certificates (Table 1) (Shepherd and Hubbard 1983). These statistics helped validate observations and support the hypothesis that a change in practice patterns had occurred in San Diego County.

Another result of the San Diego project was its impact on the quality of care. Findings indicated that the quality of care received by CHAMPUS inpatients improved.

Questionnaires were sent to psychiatrists and hospitals involved in caring for CHAMPUS inpatients after the first year of the project. Among other things, they were asked how this project had impacted patient care. Psychiatric nurse specialists in the various hospitals reported that CHAMPUS patients were now receiving better care. They said that the frequency of treatment team meetings with physicians had increased since the concurrent review program had begun. They noticed that attending physicians were conveying more information to them regarding patients' problems and instructing them on the most therapeutic ways to interact with patients. This enhanced the therapeutic ambience of the milieu portion of the treatment program and increased the number and quality of therapeutic interactions between patients and staff. The nursing staff, in turn, provided physicians with more useful data in their treatment team meetings. This significant increase in exchanging useful patient information between psychiatrist and nursing personnel was a significant factor in improving the quality of care. Nursing personnel were assigned a greater role in the treatment process and began to feel that their participation and input into the development of patients' treatment plans were valued by physicians.

## AREA OR STATE LEVEL

In addition to the peer review projects at the district branch and national levels, the area levels of the APA have also been active. One such effort, Area VI, which encompasses the state of California, should be highlighted. While diversity of opinion abounds in this area, a consensus on the importance of peer review exists. Area VI has a state peer review committee as well as a state insurance committee. Sometimes, the two have worked together. In late 1977 and early 1978, California psychiatry was presented with a challenge.

In early 1977, Ralph W. Schaffarzick, M.D., the medical director of Blue Shield of California, sent written inquiries to the California Psychiatric Association and to the Area VI Council asking if psychotherapy was still an accepted and current treatment modality. Although some felt loath to acknowledge the letter, others believed that it should be vigorously addressed. The Area VI Council asked its peer review committee to address this issue.

A six-member ad hoc committee was appointed representing the peer review committees of the four California district branches. The committee, of which I was a member, contacted Dr. Schaffarzick and lobbied for a meeting or series of meetings between representatives of Blue Shield of California and the California Psychiatric Association to address his concerns regarding the use of psychotherapy. He was a little surprised by the magnitude of the committee's response and relayed our interest in responding to their concern to the Medical Policy Committee of Blue Shield of California.

On 20 November 1977, the California Psychiatric Society Peer Review Committee voted to recommend that the medical director initiate an ad hoc committee to establish written criteria for the appropriate use of psychotherapy.

Initially, the attitude of the nonpsychiatric members of the ad hoc committee was somewhat hostile. They viewed psychiatry as having little organization and no criteria, standards, or agreement within the profession regarding psychiatric care. They were caught unprepared for our unified front and knowledge of the issues. As a result, the Area VI committee's members defused this hostile situation and gained the respect of the full ad hoc committee. We also educated the ad hoc committee about the appropriate use of psychotherapy. They eventually accepted our input. This allowed the ad hoc committee to develop criteria for the use of psychotherapy, reflecting the position of organized psychiatry.

Final recommendations were forwarded to the Medical Policy Committee (California Blue Shield). All forms of psychotherapy, from supportive to psychoanalysis, were included. The three initial criteria demonstrate the scope and impact of our peer review activities:

1. Psychiatric care benefits should be based on the same criteria as other types of medical care (i.e., medical necessity as recognized by the profession).
2. Peer review should serve the central role in determining the appropriateness of a given treatment modality in general and the appropriateness of its use in a given care.
3. Confidentiality safeguards must be carefully observed in all cases.

Specific guideline recommendations were also made.

The final result of this peer review activity came on 20 June 1979, when the committee report was accepted by the

Medical Policy Committee of Blue Shield of California. Once again, organized psychiatry had shown it could deal with the problems of third-party payers in an effective and professional way.

## NATIONAL LEVEL

Let us move on to some of the findings and results of peer review on the national level. The chapter "A Brief History of the American Psychiatric Association's Involvement in Peer Review" chronicles the development of peer review activities on the national level. The APA Committee on Peer Review and the APA National Advisory Committee (NAC) to OCHAMPUS both played leading roles.

In 1977–1979, the NAC developed standards, criteria, and peer review procedures for both inpatient and outpatient care. Before the national CHAMPUS review program was operational, the system was given a trial run. Hospital care in excess of 180 days was evaluated using NAC criteria. The cases were reviewed by psychiatrists in the geographical areas where treatment was rendered. This was the first review of psychiatric care on a national level since the Select Committee on Psychiatric Care and Evaluation (SCOPCE) I committee had reviewed CHAMPUS residential treatment center care in 1975. Reviewers' findings and recommendations were carefully evaluated by the NAC. The reviewers' decisions were based on issues of documented medical necessity and appropriateness of treatment provided in each case, as well as the patients' ability to respond to treatment.

The results of the trial run were striking and the professionalism exhibited by the reviewers was generally laudable. Furthermore, OCHAMPUS was also pleased with the results. Thus, in October 1980 the national review program for CHAMPUS began, although several months passed before it became fully operational. Over the last several years, this program has been under constant evaluation and many of the problems have been overcome. The NAC works at improving the system.

There is an ongoing effort to educate the APA membership regarding peer review concepts and their application. For example, Continuing Medical Education workshops on peer review have been held at the APA annual meeting, as well as forums on peer review. In addition, the director of the Office of Peer Review, Peer Review Committee members, and key staff have traveled around the country to area councils and district branch meetings to discuss peer review issues and to present status reports and findings on the APA's peer review projects. The feedback from the membership of the APA and its district branches has played a vital role in refining peer review concepts and in developing procedures and instruments such as the peer review questionnaire.

There are several Blue Cross/Blue Shield Plans that act as the fiscal intermediaries (FIs) for OCHAMPUS. They contract with OCHAMPUS to perform claims processing services for various geographic areas of the country. As a result, they play a central role in the administration of the review project. Periodically, the FI for one area may change because the contracts are awarded on a competitive basis. The education of the FIs is also one of the APA's most important jobs. The fact that there are several different FIs complicates this effort because each organization has its own strengths and weaknesses. Overall coordination has nonetheless reached a professional level.

The data presented in Table 2, from OCHAMPUS fiscal year 1982 (1 October 1981, to 1 October 1982), give some statistical information on the project (Altman H, personal communications, 21 November 1980).

**Table 2.** OCHAMPUS Data for Fiscal Year 1982

| Cases Reviewed by Peer Review | Inpatient | | Outpatient | |
|---|---|---|---|---|
| | N | % | N | % |
| Approved | 2448 | 60 | 2433 | 53 |
| Partially approved | 1078 | 27 | 1763 | 38 |
| Denied | 526 | 13 | 419 | 9 |
| Total | 4052 | 100 | 4615 | 100 |

As peer review continues, I expect to see the percentage of denials decrease, particularly as providers improve their documentation. Additionally, the small segment of providers who overutilize or give substandard care will either drop from the system or improve their utilization or quality of care.

OCHAMPUS statistics for fiscal year 1982 indicate that while medical-surgical costs increased 35 percent, costs for the total mental health benefit (which includes all other mental health professions) rose 20 percent during that time. Alex Rodriguez, M.D., medical director of OCHAMPUS, has stated that this represents, at the most conservative estimate, a savings of approximately $5 million (Business and Health 1984).

In his conversations with Norman Penner, APA Peer Review project director, Allen McLean, M.D., a psychiatrist at IBM, indicated that during 1981 −1982, IBM's mental health costs increased 35 percent (as did medical surgical costs). At this writing, IBM has no peer review system. This makes CHAMPUS' figures even more meaningful.

William Guillette, M.D., then the medical director of Aetna, indicated a savings for Aetna of some 3 percent during the first full year of operating their APA peer review programs (Guillette W, presentation before APA Peer Review Committee, Washington, DC, 1981). The previous year they paid out approximately $89 million for mental health benefits. Aetna was impressed and pleased by this savings of $2.7 million.

Robert Long, M.D., the medical director of Mutual of Omaha, reported that for calendar year 1982, their first full year of using APAs peer review system, they saved $200,000–$300,000. This savings cost them just under $10,000, based on only 69 peer review cases.

The private insurance sector feels that they also reduce costs through peer review's sentinel effect, as well as by the review process itself. They generally send only a small percentage of cases to the APA for peer review.

The private insurance sector as well as OCHAMPUS had relatively little statistical data on claims paid prior to the use of peer review. Consequently, we are still short on hard statistical data. The greatest indicator of the APA peer review program's effectiveness is that at this writing, 27 additional private insurance companies have purchased peer review services. They also feel that the peer review process upgrades the quality of care in addition to reducing costs.

Representatives from OCHAMPUS and the private insurance sector have met with the APA Peer Review Committee during its fall business meetings for the past several years. In the beginning, the insurers were reserved and

tentative in their comments. However, they became increasingly impressed with the professionalism and knowledge of the committee. They were especially impressed with
the committee's understanding of the insurance industry's
fears and concerns about psychiatric benefits. They came to
see that we were willing to agree that there are problems and
we were ready to deal with those problems actively. The
APA's *Manual of Psychiatric Peer Review* (1980) and DSM-
III (1981) represent standards, guidelines, and criteria
unique in medicine. In fact, the insurance companies and
OCHAMPUS now feel that the APA has developed a peer
review capability that serves as a model for what they would
like to see in the rest of medicine.

It is of interest that Aetna has increased the mental
health benefits they now offer their own employees. Additionally, a very large employer is considering an expansion
of benefits on a case-by-case basis when medical necessity
is present as determined by peer review. At this time of
recession and cutbacks, these two items are of significance.

There is a further result of the APA's peer review activities that should be addressed. Because OCHAMPUS was
pleased with the "San Diego experience," they asked that
standards and criteria for the review of residential treatment centers for children and adolescents be developed.
They then asked that these guidelines be used to review
three residential treatment centers in San Diego County for
a pilot peer review project. Subsequently, the standards and
criteria developed in San Diego were used as a basis for
developing CHAMPUS' national criteria for residential treatment centers. These national standards helped preserve the
care of these centers as a covered CHAMPUS benefit.

In addition, OCHAMPUS asked the NAC to develop
standards and criteria to define and review partial hospital
care. These criteria may soon result in partial hospital care
or day treatment as a new CHAMPUS benefit.

Peer review has identified problem providers, including
hospitals and individual psychiatrists. In some cases, this
resulted in face-to-face discussions of the apparent problems between the individual provider of care and a member
of the NAC. These discussions were usually productive and
resolved the problems.

Problem hospitals may be subject to on-site visits by
OCHAMPUS and a clinical team consisting of psychiatrists,

psychologists, and a psychiatric nurse specialist. These on-site visits are for the purpose of determining the quality and appropriateness of care provided by the facilities. On-site visits result in significant changes in the program offered and the nature and quality of documentation of that care.

Aetna and OCHAMPUS made it clear that if peer review did not yield its expected outcomes, they would make major cuts in mental health benefits. The peer review activities of the APA at the district branch and national level have played a central role in maintaining third-party participation in covering mental health care. Without that participation, the practice of psychiatry as we know it today would not exist.

## REFERENCES

American Psychiatric Association: Diagnostic and Statistical Manual of Mental Disorders, 3rd ed. Washington, DC, American Psychiatric Association, 1980

American Psychiatric Association: Manual of Psychiatric Peer Review, 2nd ed. Washington, DC, American Psychiatric Association, 1981

Peer review program sets trends in claims processing. Business and Health 1:21–25, 1984

Shepherd G, Hubbard B. Statistical Analysis and Evaluation of the Concurrent Psychiatric Review Project: San Diego Psychiatric Society (DOD Contract No. MDA 906-83-C-0002). Aurora, Colorado, Office of Civilian Health and Medical Program of the Uniformed Services, 1983

# 12

# Promise

*John M. Hamilton, M.D.*

# Promise

The promise of peer review epitomizes how the ideal peer review program should work to attain an ideal set of goals for patients, providers, and third-party payers.

Ideally, a peer review process should be a part of a broad-based quality assurance effort that includes, but is not necessarily limited to, case management services, preadmission screening, and authorization and utilization review. The peer review program should have prospective, concurrent, and retrospective review capabilities. It should have direct access to research and educational components.

As stated elsewhere in this book, medical systems' architecture and economics are constantly changing. The ideal quality assurance system will change with them to insist that the patient receives the best quality medical care with the least squandering of resources. Obsolescence occurs so easily in this business. We have seen prospective payment systems, for example, make length-of-stay criteria and analysis obsolete as parameters for reimbursement, although they remained useful as tools to help assess cost effectiveness and possibly treatment efficacy. The ideal quality assurance effort has as a landmark its capacity for flexibility.

Peer review in psychiatry originated as an alternative to having insurers of health care benefits set arbitrary caps or limits on mental health services that would be reimbursed for eligible beneficiaries. This was a way for the profession to chart its own destiny with the setting of reasonable standards of care and the monitoring of service provision to detect and avoid abuse and unacceptable patterns of practice. Somehow, along with this idea, the notion of an expectation that peer review would produce an enhancement of the benefit structure began to be broadly popular among the rank and file of organized psychiatry. In discussing the ideal peer review process, we must differentiate between that process as it stands alone and that process as it lends itself to becoming one of the principal tools, if not the principal tool, of the profession's marketing strategy.

Peer review in and of itself does not and will not necessarily produce enhanced psychiatric benefits. The profession has established as an intermediate-range goal that psychiatric benefits be brought into consonance with the benefit structure for the remainder of medicine. The argument is made that the whole person should be insured against the possibility of catastrophic invasion by all manners of diseases and that to discriminate against any one of the body systems that might be invaded is intolerable in a logical and consistent world. Herein lies the ethical dilemma for medicine in the 1980s, 1990s, and in the twenty-first century.

The profession's goal of parity for all medical benefits, including benefits for mental illness, can only be achieved through a vigorous marketing strategy that uses national and local resources to influence insurers, employers, consumers, and administrators of programs. Although it is seldom mentioned in the same breath with those in the previous sentence, it is just as important to influence the providers of health care services outside the realm of mental health. It is frequently the lack of understanding on the part of these providers that breeds the hostility and adversity that negatively reinforces the doubt in the minds of executives of insurance companies and in industry who must make the vital decisions about benefits packages. What does all this have to do with the ideal peer review process as a part of the ideal quality assurance program?

The most frequent question asked by the executive when discussions about parity of benefits arise is "How can we be assured that the quality will be worth what we pay for it and how can we guard against runaway costs?" A broad-based quality assurance program of which peer review is an integral part essentially provides the mechanisms for monitoring quality and utilization and fueling the educational processes necessary for corrective and informational feedback to the on-line professional.

The ideal quality assurance program has the built-in capacity to assess trends in patterns of health care delivery and to match them with evolving reimbursement schemes so that it may develop methodologies prospectively to provide the monitoring and educational components required. A great deal of this trend assessment comes about through systematic research using the volumes of data amassed through the review efforts. It would seem useful to accommodate this massive volume of data to specific studies designed to answer some of the significant questions about cost effectiveness and treatment efficacy in psychiatric practice. Studies regarding the latter have been largely nonexistent and studies regarding the former have been sparse. An ingredient that has been lacking in the collection of data for peer review is discharge information. Detailed discharge data will have to be a part of our information arsenal if proper outcome studies are to be conducted. The studies should allow us to compare therapeutic modalities and establish reliability coefficients that should help in the determination of reasonable standards for assessment of practice patterns. These studies could also be used to validate or invalidate certain modalities that have inherent controversial concerns associated with them. A forward-looking marketing strategy has the quality assurance mechanisms and scope of review services as the backup to its lobbying for benefits enhancement. We must keep in mind, however, that it is aggressive marketing at every level that accomplishes increases in benefit; quality assurance helps maintain that achievement.

In the future, it seems that far fewer psychiatric patients will be treated as inpatients and those who are so treated will have rather markedly decreased numbers of inpatient days. (This is also true for general medical and surgical problems.) The push toward a decreased use of the inpatient bed will mean that increasing numbers of patients will get their care in outpatient or partial hospital settings and that the majority of these patients in each of the settings will be sicker and more difficult to manage. Peer review will, therefore, have to accommodate its methodologies to this change in degree of patient difficulty for all settings and will particularly have to construct review mechanisms that can respond more immediately than in the past. The use of electronic transmittal of data from provider to the review hub is one of the adjustments that will be seen. This faster turn around time will be dictated by the need to screen and preauthorize all non-emergency inpatient admissions, provide 24- to 48-hour authorization for emergency admissions, manage concurrent monitoring of all inpatient stays, and give authorization for transfers to alternative level of care settings. Much more dependence will be placed on the "hub" of review operations, with exceptionally well-qualified clinical coordinating personnel serving as the conduit among provider, third-party payer, and peer review so that rapid, maximally informed decision making can occur.

A brief look at some of the details of the system of the future described in the foregoing paragraph and a look at how a national specialty society might cope with and overcome the problems accompanying the implementation of such a method is necessary here.

Fortunately, technology has provided the electronic capacity to communicate data across the vast expanse of our nation almost instantaneously no matter the location, urban or rural. There will, nonetheless, have to be skilled clinicians at the terminals to receive as well as transmit the data. These professionals and the network of local consultants established in each state or region are the keys to a successful system for rapid preadmission certification and concurrent monitoring of inpatient stays. Providers of service must have immediate access to reviewers and certifiers, and authorizers must have immediate access to insurers and employer's claims processors, facilities, and attendings. Telecommunications equipment will obviously facilitate this access. This freedom of access presupposes an attitude of trust and mutual respect that must exist between the communicating parties.

A national specialty society must decide on an organization structure to abet the kind of communication system discussed and to provide the environment within which the process can grow. For psychiatry there are two alternatives that seem to stand out among several. A quality assurance division might be established within the American Psychiatric Association (APA), with quasi-autonomy to carry out the functions related to preadmission authorization, concurrent review, and other case-management services including peer review. The APA might also create a wholly owned subsidiary (either a profit or nonprofit corporation) that might be chartered to carry out these activities independently. The latter might have a slight advantage over the former in competing against other entities and agencies seeking to provide similar services. Either structure would have the capacity or entities spawned by them by agreements of understanding or subcontracts to conduct the local aspects of the business when this seemed desirable.

The emergence of preadmission screening and authorization for most admissions in medicine as a whole, and for a considerable number of psychiatric admissions as well, and the need to establish controls for inpatient stays will make the development of accurate utilization review criteria invaluable in the mounting of a serious quality assurance effort for psychiatry. Developing reasonable national utilization review criteria from the myriad divergent local criteria currently in existence may indeed be one of psychiatry's paramount challenges of this decade.

The demise of Professional Standards Review Organizations (PSROs) and the birth of Peer Review Organizations (PROs) dictated by the Social Security Amendments of 1983 (PL98-21) deserve attention here as a part of the evolutionary process in the development of quality assurance programming for the health care industry.

The shift from a cost-based, retrospective reimbursement system as the method of payment for medicare inpatient hospitalization to a Prospective Payment System based on diagnosis-related groups mandated a new system to monitor the quality of care and its cost effectiveness. The Health Care Financial Administration (HCFA) of the Social Security Administration was empowered to contract with PROs in 54 locals (all states, some territories, and the District of Columbia) to provide health care monitoring services for Medicare beneficiaries. Specifically, these PROs were to agree to a management-by-objectives system to validate their existence. These objectives fall in the categories of admission and procedure objectives and quality objectives. The key word in these objectives is *reduction*. The PRO must agree in advance to reduce numbers of admissions involving care that could be given on an ambulatory basis and care that would be considered inappropriate or unnecessary by local and regional standards. The quality objectives are also stated in "reduction" terms related to ratiogenic complications, unnecessary surgery, avoidable deaths, etc. Specific activities are required of the PRO to carry out its mission; the numerical objectives in the reduction areas would be considered obligatory for renewal of the contract with HCFA. This may seem somewhat harsh, but accountability has become more than just a watchword in the 1980s. It is an action word. This new reimbursement system and the monitoring system that accompanies it should provide psychiatry with the insights necessary to help resculpt its own quality assurance effort with an equally creative spirit.

In an appearance before the U.S. Senate Subcommittee on Health (Committee on Finance 7/31/84), Dr. Caroline K. Davis, HCFA administrator, said:

> In order to assure that high quality patient care continues to be provided to our beneficiaries, the Congress put a strong mechanism in place to assure that quality is maintained. We believe that the vast majority of physicians and hospitals will continue to provide high quality and appropriate care. However, it is our responsibility to assure that this is the case. Each PRO will be obligated to conduct meaningful quality review and achieve significant impact on the quality of care furnished to Medicare beneficiaries in its area. We believe that the PROs can meet this challenge and become an integral part of the nation's total health care system. . . . Thus I assure you: The HCFA has set a high priority on developing and implementing an effective medical review system which will examine both the cost and quality of care.

Organized psychiatry can afford no less a priority nor commitment to its quality assurance programming.

# EDUCATION

An attitude of learning should exist for a lifetime. Those of us who have entered a profession should carry an attitude of teaching—learning throughout the course of our professional practice. Peer review, ideally, is built around just such a conceptualization. Essentially, this was the system of learning with which we were involved during our clinical clerkship years in medical school, during our internships and residencies, and during any postresidency fellowships with which we were associated. Peer review is a continuation of the same process. It also follows the precepts of quality assurance programming where (1) appropriate performance standards that can be suitably measured are set, (2) a method of monitoring that performance is established, (3) a system of feedback for deficient performance as well as for efficient and effective performance is initiated, and (4) methods to maintain quality performance once it is attained are in place.

Educational and administrative strategies provide the methods by which informational and corrective feedback are made available to on-line clinicians in the field. In the future, specific programs will be constructed using state-of-the-art audio and video techniques to allow practitioners to hear and/or see their performance evaluated and critiqued in their office, home, or car by direct telephone transmission or by tape or disc.

Earlier it was indicated that the ideal peer review system must be attached to an educational component. This is the hookup necessary to make certain that findings about the quality of provider performance that do not meet the standard of care required can be transformed into attractive educational programming that can be used by the provider to buoy knowledge in the discovered area of below-standard performance. This, of course, is the preferred method of achieving performance change. Administrative actions such as payment cutoffs or removal from rosters of providers eligible to give services are not the best means to achieve change among professionals. These sanctions would, of course, only be used against the provider who exhibited continuous poor performance while remaining recalcitrant to the educational approach. Peer review is, after all, essentially an educational process.

## RESEARCH

Psychiatry has been most lax in engaging in efficacy of therapy research; this is most pronounced in the areas of interpersonal therapies and in long-term hospitalization for intensive intervention designed to treat chronic, severely disabled psychiatric patients, with the goal of restructuring the personality. The tremendous amounts of data collected during the course of careful quality assurance programming (which includes peer review) will lend itself to thoughtful research that could shed some light in the efficacy of therapy area. To do this effectively, peer review must, as earlier stated, be attached to a research component.

Any effective program must be capable of evaluating its own performance. This is as important for peer review as for any other. A research component would enhance the program's self-evaluative capacity with protocols structured from the outset to test quality assurance's effectiveness and efficiency. The question of "who monitors the monitor?" is always a difficult one. This capacity will be built into the quality assurance program of the future.

A research component can also be charged with monitoring the program's security in regard to both its internal operational processes and its external relationships. The concern about confidentiality, which is always forward in this work, can be strongly diminished by a sophisticated research component's guards over the program's security. Program security will become more and more sophisticated and important as our systems become more electronically driven.

## THE PEER REVIEWER

The peer reviewer remains and will remain the critical element in the peer review process. So much depends on the method of selection, the credentialing, the validation of credentials, the orientation and continuing education of the reviewer, the responsiveness of the reviewer to the standards and their interpretation, the reviewer's universal understanding of what constitutes medical necessity and what acceptable intervention modalities are, and the willingness to communicate with peers in reporting findings in a professional, erudite, yet compassionate fashion, particularly when deficits are detected.

All of these areas have been discussed as concerns in another chapter of this book. How will we address these issues in the future? Some would say that political, ideological, and logistical difficulties grossly hamper our capacity and our will to do anything constructive about them. Despite the barricades, we must resolve these issues, some of which have confronted us as impasses for decades.

The whole question of "who is a peer" will be resolved by the creation of coalitions that might have seemed impossible in the past. Many of us have become so unique in our own eyes as to say we have no peers. If one has no peer, how can proficiency be measured? That becomes a very important consideration. In the future, we will work out internal professional systems linking our training programs of all varieties to national and local licensing and certification centers, which will allow certification of specific credentials for all practicing professionals. This local and national credentialing system will produce computer-correlated lists of peers for every operation in which we engage clinically, and this listing will give us our rosters of certified peers for every possible clinical situation. Computers, however, are only able to spew forth that for which they have been programmed using accurate data input. The responsibility for those programs and data are ours as professionals. We must resolve our parochial differences to allow this process to occur rationally.

## SUMMARY

Peer review must be seen, as we have known it, as a primordial step toward the total quality assurance programming of the future. Quality assurance will be composed of a brace of services that will include preadmission screening and certification of all non-emergency inpatient admissions, early authorization (within the first 24 to 48 hours) for all other admissions, and case-management services (monitoring the remainder of the inpatient stay and authorizing transfers to alternate levels of care, residential or outpatient). Quality of provider performance will be the commodity assessed. Quality assurance programming will have sophisticated educational and research areas to provide the feedback of findings to practitioners and to develop some of the answers about our efficiency and effectiveness, which have gone unanswered too long. We must continue to emphasize the importance of the peer reviewer in this process. The selection, the training, and the quality of the reviewer are the essential ingredients of a viable program. The electronic age, with the burst of technology surrounding it, makes these processes easier than ever before.

   We must renew our dedication to excellence in the art and science of medicine. We must insist on radically extricating mediocrity from ourselves and our colleagues. We must insist on precision and compassion as we perfervidly use our clinical and administrative skills for the benefit of our patients. We must guard against the subtle seductions that tempt us to convert more and more of the nation's health care expenditures into health care incomes. The ideal quality assurance programming will be designed to monitor these performances. We can meet the challenge and have a vital part in its design and implementation, or we can decline the challenge and have it done for or to us. I think that we have demonstrated that we can meet the challenge and that we can best serve our patients and colleagues when we do.

# Index